T0362395

# Imaging of the Mediastinum

*Editor*

## BRETT W. CARTER

# RADIOLOGIC CLINICS OF NORTH AMERICA

www.radiologic.theclinics.com

*Consulting Editor*
## FRANK H. MILLER

March 2021 • Volume 59 • Number 2

**ELSEVIER**

1600 John F. Kennedy Boulevard • Suite 1800 • Philadelphia, Pennsylvania, 19103-2899

http://www.theclinics.com

**RADIOLOGIC CLINICS OF NORTH AMERICA Volume 59, Number 2**
**March 2021 ISSN 0033-8389, ISBN 13: 978-0-323-76272-4**

Editor: John Vassallo (j.vassallo@elsevier.com)
Developmental Editor: Karen Justine Solomon

**© 2021 Elsevier Inc. All rights reserved.**

This periodical and the individual contributions contained in it are protected under copyright by Elsevier, and the following terms and conditions apply to their use:

**Photocopying**
Single photocopies of single articles may be made for personal use as allowed by national copyright laws. Permission of the Publisher and payment of a fee is required for all other photocopying, including multiple or systematic copying, copying for advertising or promotional purposes, resale, and all forms of document delivery. Special rates are available for educational institutions that wish to make photocopies for non-profit educational classroom use. For information on how to seek permission visit www.elsevier.com/permissions or call: (+44) 1865 843830 (UK)/(+1) 215 239 3804 (USA).

**Derivative Works**
Subscribers may reproduce tables of contents or prepare lists of articles including abstracts for internal circulation within their institutions. Permission of the Publisher is required for resale or distribution outside the institution. Permission of the Publisher is required for all other derivative works, including compilations and translations (please consult www.elsevier.com/permissions).

**Electronic Storage or Usage**
Permission of the Publisher is required to store or use electronically any material contained in this periodical, including any article or part of an article (please consult www.elsevier.com/permissions). Except as outlined above, no part of this publication may be reproduced, stored in a retrieval system or transmitted in any form or by any means, electronic, mechanical, photocopying, recording or otherwise, without prior written permission of the Publisher.

**Notice**
No responsibility is assumed by the Publisher for any injury and/or damage to persons or property as a matter of products liability, negligence or otherwise, or from any use or operation of any methods, products, instructions or ideas contained in the material herein. Because of rapid advances in the medical sciences, in particular, independent verification of diagnoses and drug dosages should be made.

Although all advertising material is expected to conform to ethical (medical) standards, inclusion in this publication does not constitute a guarantee or endorsement of the quality or value of such product or of the claims made of it by its manufacturer.

*Radiologic Clinics of North America* (ISSN 0033-8389) is published bimonthly by Elsevier Inc., 360 Park Avenue South, New York, NY 10010-1710. Months of issue are January, March, May, July, September, and November. Periodicals postage paid at New York, NY and additional mailing offices. Subscription prices are USD 518 per year for US individuals, USD 1309 per year for US institutions, USD 100 per year for US students and residents, USD 611 per year for Canadian individuals, USD 1368 per year for Canadian institutions, USD 703 per year for international individuals, USD 1368 per year for international institutions, USD 100 per year for Canadian students/residents, and USD 315 per year for international students/residents. To receive student and resident rate, orders must be accompanied by name of affiliated institution, date of term and the signature of program/residency coordinatior on institution letterhead. Orders will be billed at individual rate until proof of status is received. Foreign air speed delivery is included in all *Clinics* subscription prices. All prices are subject to change without notice. **POSTMASTER:** Send address changes to *Radiologic Clinics of North America*, Elsevier Health Sciences Division, Subscription Customer Service, 3251 Riverport Lane, Maryland Heights, MO63043. **Customer Service: Telephone: 1-800-654-2452** (U.S. and Canada); **1-314-447-8871** (outside U.S. and Canada). **Fax: 1-314-447-8029. E-mail: journalscustomerservice-usa@elsevier.com (for print support); journalsonlinesupport-usa@elsevier.com (for online support)**.

*Reprints.* For copies of 100 or more of articles in this publication, please contact the Commercial Reprints Department, Elsevier Inc., 360 Park Avenue South, New York, New York 10010-1710. Tel.: +1-212-633-3874; Fax: +1-212-633-3820; E-mail: reprints@elsevier.com.

*Radiologic Clinics of North America* also published in Greek Paschalidis Medical Publications, Athens, Greece.

*Radiologic Clinics of North America* is covered in *MEDLINE/PubMed (Index Medicus), EMBASE/Excerpta Medica, Current Contents/Life Sciences, Current Contents/Clinical Medicine, RSNA Index to Imaging Literature, BIOSIS, Science Citation Index,* and *ISI/BIOMED.*

# Contributors

## CONSULTING EDITOR

**FRANK H. MILLER, MD, FACR**
Lee F. Rogers MD Professor of Medical Education, Chief, Body Imaging Section and Fellowship Program, Medical Director, MRI, Department of Radiology, Northwestern Memorial Hospital, Northwestern University, Feinberg School of Medicine, Chicago, Illinois, USA

## EDITOR

**BRETT W. CARTER, MD**
Director of Clinical Operations, Chief Patient Safety and Quality Officer, Diagnostic Imaging, Associate Professor, Department of Thoracic Imaging, The University of Texas MD Anderson Cancer Center, Houston, Texas, USA

## AUTHORS

**FEREIDOUN ABTIN, MD**
Professor of Radiology, Thoracic and Interventional Section, Department of Radiological Sciences, David Geffen School of Medicine at UCLA, Los Angeles, California, USA

**JEANNE B. ACKMAN, MD, FACR**
Assistant Professor of Radiology, Harvard Medical School, Director of Thoracic MRI, Division of Thoracic Imaging and Intervention, Department of Radiology, Massachusetts General Hospital, Boston, Massachusetts, USA

**SADIQ ALQUTUB, MD**
Department of Pathology, The George Washington University Hospital, Washington, DC, USA

**ELENA BEKKER, MD**
Department of Diagnostic Imaging, Divisions of Cardiovascular Imaging and Thoracic Imaging, The Chaim Sheba Medical Center (affiliated with Tel Aviv University), Tel Aviv, Ramat Gan, Israel

**MARCELO F.K. BENVENISTE, MD**
Associate Professor, Thoracic Imaging Department, The University of Texas MD Anderson Cancer Center, Houston, Texas, USA

**SONIA L. BETANCOURT-CUELLAR, MD**
Associate Professor, Thoracic Imaging Department, Division of Diagnostic Imaging, The University of Texas MD Anderson Cancer Center, Houston, Texas, USA

**DAVID M. BIKO, MD**
Director of Pediatric Cardiovascular and Lymphatic Imaging, Department of Radiology, Children's Hospital of Philadelphia, University of Pennsylvania Perelman School of Medicine, Philadelphia, Pennsylvania, USA

**PATRICK P. BOURGOUIN, MD, FRCPC**
Clinical Fellow, Department of Radiology,
Brigham and Women's Hospital, Boston,
Massachusetts, USA

**BRETT W. CARTER, MD**
Director of Clinical Operations, Chief Patient
Safety and Quality Officer, Diagnostic
Imaging, Associate Professor, Department of
Thoracic Imaging, The University of Texas MD
Anderson Cancer Center, Houston, Texas,
USA

**ADAM R. DULBERGER, MD, Capt, USAF,
MC**
Department of Radiology, David Grant
Medical Center, Travis Air Force Base,
California, USA

**DANE A. FISHER, MD, Capt, USAF**
Department of Radiology, Naval Medical
Center Portsmouth, Portsmouth, Virginia,
USA

**SHERIEF H. GARRANA, MD**
Thoracic Radiologist, Department of
Radiology, Saint Luke's Hospital of Kansas
City, Assistant Professor of Radiology,
University of Missouri-Kansas City School of
Medicine, Kansas City, Missouri, USA

**ORLY GOITEIN, MD**
Assistant Professor of Radiology,
Department of Diagnostic Imaging,
Division of Cardiovascular Imaging, The
Chaim Sheba Medical Center (affiliated with
Tel Aviv University), Tel Aviv, Ramat Gan,
Israel

**ALLEN P. HEEGER, DO**
Department of Radiology, Division of Thoracic
Imaging and Intervention, Harvard Medical
School, Massachusetts General Hospital,
Boston, Massachusetts, USA

**WAYNE L. HOFSTETTER, MD**
Professor, Cardiothoracic Department, The
University of Texas MD Anderson Cancer
Center, Houston, Texas, USA

**SOHEIL KOORAKI, MD**
Fellow, Department of Nuclear Medicine,
University of California, Los Angeles (UCLA),
Los Angeles, California, USA

**JOHN P. LICHTENBERGER III, MD**
Associate Professor and Chief of Thoracic
Imaging, Department of Radiology, The
George Washington University Medical Faculty
Associates, Washington, DC, USA

**RACHNA MADAN, MD**
Associate Staff Radiologist, Division of
Thoracic Imaging, Assistant Professor,
Department of Radiology, Brigham and
Women's Hospital, Harvard Medical School,
Boston, Massachusetts, USA

**MARIA A. MANNING, MD**
GI Section Chief and Associate Physician in
Chief, American Institute for Radiologic
Pathology, American College of Radiology,
Silver Spring, MD and Associate Professor,
MedStar Georgetown University Hospital,
Washington, DC, USA

**EDITH M. MAROM, MD**
Professor of Radiology, Department of
Diagnostic Imaging, Division of Thoracic
Imaging, The Chaim Sheba Medical Center
(affiliated with Tel Aviv University), Tel Aviv,
Ramat Gan, Israel

**DIANA P. PALACIO, MD**
Associate Professor, Department of Medical
Imaging, The University of Arizona - Banner
Medical Center, Tucson, Arizona, USA

**REGINA F. PARKER, MA/MBA**
Harvard Medical School, Boston,
Massachusetts, USA

**MICHAEL A. PAVIO, MD**
Department of Radiology, Walter Reed
National Military Medical Center, Bethesda,
Maryland, USA

**P. GABRIEL PETERSON, MD, LTC, USA**
Chief of Cardiothoracic Imaging, Department
of Radiology, Walter Reed National Military
Medical Center, Bethesda, Maryland, USA

**MELISSA L. ROSADO-DE-CHRISTENSON, MD, FACR**
Chief of Thoracic Imaging, Department of Radiology, Saint Luke's Hospital of Kansas City, Professor of Radiology, University of Missouri-Kansas City School of Medicine, Kansas City, Missouri, USA

**CHAD D. STRANGE, MD**
Division of Diagnostic Imaging, The University of Texas MD Anderson Cancer Center, Houston, Texas, USA

**MYLENE T. TRUONG, MD**
Professor of Radiology, Department of Diagnostic Imaging, Division of Thoracic Imaging, The University of Texas MD Anderson Cancer Center, Houston, Texas, USA

**MERISSA N. ZEMAN, MD**
Department of Radiology, The George Washington University Hospital, Washington, DC, USA

# Contents

Numerous systems have been created to divide the mediastinum into specific compartments for the purposes of generating a focused differential diagnosis for masses and other abnormalities identified on imaging, planning for biopsies and surgical interventions, and facilitating communication between health care professionals in a multidisciplinary setting. Most have focused on imaging and are based on arbitrary landmarks delineated on the lateral chest radiograph. The International Thymic Malignancy Interest Group has developed a classification system based on cross-sectional imaging, defining specific prevascular, visceral, and paravertebral compartments, that has been accepted as a new standard and is the topic of this review.

Prevascular mediastinal masses include a wide range of benign and malignant entities. Localization of mediastinal masses to specific compartments together with characteristic imaging findings and demographic and clinical information allows formulation of a focused differential diagnosis. Radiologists may use these methods to distinguish between surgical and nonsurgical cases and thus inform patient management and have an impact on outcomes. Treatment of choice varies based on the pathology, ranging from no intervention or serial imaging follow-up to surgical excision, chemotherapy, and/or radiation.

Thymic epithelial neoplasms, as classified by the World Health Organization, include thymoma, thymic carcinoma, and thymic carcinoid. They are a rare group of tumors and are often diagnosed incidentally in the work-up of parathymic syndrome, such as myasthenia gravis, or when mass effect or local invasion causes other symptoms. In each of these scenarios, understanding the radiologic-pathologic relationship of these tumors allows clinical imagers to contribute meaningfully to management decisions and overall patient care. Integrating important imaging features, such as local invasion, and pathologic features, such as necrosis and immunohistochemistry, ensures a meaningful contribution by clinical imagers to the care team.

Thymic epithelial neoplasms are a group of malignant tumors that includes thymoma, thymic carcinoma, and thymic neuroendocrine tumors. Although several staging systems have been developed over the years for use with these cancers, they have been interpreted and implemented in a nonuniform manner. Recently, the International Association for the study of Lung Cancer and the International Thymic Malignancy Interest Group developed a tumor-node-metastasis staging system that has been universally accepted and correlates with patient survival and outcomes. Although pathologic staging is determined by histologic examination of the resected tumor, imaging plays an important role in clinical staging and is important for informing therapeutic decisions.

The visceral mediastinum contains important vascular and non-vascular structures including the heart, great vessels, lymph nodes, and portions of the esophagus and trachea. Multiple imaging modalities, including chest radiography, computed tomography, MR imaging, and nuclear medicine studies, can be used to detect, diagnose, and characterize masses in this compartment. Lymphadenopathy is the most common process involving the visceral mediastinum and can be seen with a wide variety of diseases. Less commonly seen entities include foregut duplication cysts, neoplasms and other lesions arising from the trachea and esophagus, paragangliomas as well as other mesenchymal tumors.

The epidemiology and clinical management of esophageal carcinomas are changing, and clinical imagers are required to understand both the imaging appearances of common cancers and the pathologic diagnoses that drive management. Rare esophageal malignancies and benign esophageal neoplasms have distinct imaging features that may suggest a diagnosis and guide the next steps clinically. Furthermore, these imaging features have a basis in pathology, and this article focuses on the relationship between pathologic features and imaging manifestations that will help an informed imager maintain clinical relevance.

Esophageal cancer is an uncommon malignancy that ranks sixth in terms of mortality worldwide. Squamous cell carcinoma is the predominant histologic subtype worldwide whereas adenocarcinoma represents the majority of cases in North America, Australia, and Europe. Esophageal cancer is staged using the American Joint Committee on Cancer and the International Union for Cancer Control TNM system and has separate classifications for the clinical, pathologic, and postneoadjuvant pathologic stage groups. The determination of clinical TNM is based on complementary imaging modalities, including esophagogastroduodenoscopy/endoscopic ultrasound; endoscopic ultrasound–fine-needle aspiration; computed tomography of the chest, abdomen, and pelvis; and fluorodeoxyglucose PET/computed tomography.

Soheil Kooraki and Fereidoun Abtin

Optimal assessment of the mediastinal masses is performed by a combination of clinical, radiological and often histological assessments. Image-guided transthoracic biopsy of mediastinal lesions is a minimally invasive and reliable procedure to obtain tissue samples, establish a diagnosis and provide a treatment plan. Biopsy can be performed under Computed Tomography, MRI, or ultrasound guidance, using a fine needle aspiration or a core-needle. In this paper, we review the image-guided strategies and techniques for histologic sampling of mediastinal lesions, along with the related clinical scenarios and possible procedural complications. In addition, image-guided mediastinal drainage and mediastinal ablations will be briefly discussed.

## PROGRAM OBJECTIVE

The objective of the *Radiologic Clinics of North America* is to keep practicing radiologists and radiology residents up to date with current clinical practice in radiology by providing timely articles reviewing the state of the art in patient care.

## TARGET AUDIENCE

Practicing radiologists, radiology residents, and other healthcare professionals who provide patient care utilizing radiologic findings.

## LEARNING OBJECTIVES

Upon completion of this activity, participants will be able to:
1. Describe the details of the tumor-node-metastasis (TNM) staging systems for such cancers as esophageal cancer and thymic epithelial neoplasms.
2. Discuss the radiologic-pathologic correlation articles between imaging findings, staging systems, and histopathologic analysis.
3. Recognize the role of MR imaging in the evaluation of mediastinal abnormalities, potential pitfalls in evaluating mediastinal masses, and the methods used by interventional radiologists to biopsy and treat mediastinal lesions.

## ACCREDITATION

The Elsevier Office of Continuing Medical Education (EOCME) is accredited by the Accreditation Council for Continuing Medical Education (ACCME) to provide continuing medical education for physicians.

The EOCME designates this journal-based CME activity for a maximum of 12 *AMA PRA Category 1 Credit*(s)™. Physicians should claim only the credit commensurate with the extent of their participation in the activity.

All other healthcare professionals requesting continuing education credit for this enduring material will be issued a certificate of participation.

## DISCLOSURE OF CONFLICTS OF INTEREST

The EOCME assesses conflict of interest with its instructors, faculty, planners, and other individuals who are in a position to control the content of CME activities. All relevant conflicts of interest that are identified are thoroughly vetted by EOCME for fair balance, scientific objectivity, and patient care recommendations. EOCME is committed to providing its learners with CME activities that promote improvements or quality in healthcare and not a specific proprietary business or a commercial interest.

**The planning committee, staff, authors and editors listed below have identified no financial relationships or relationships to products or devices they or their spouse/life partner have with commercial interest related to the content of this CME activity:**
Fereidoun Abtin, MD; Jeanne B. Ackman, MD, FACR; Sadiq Alqutub, MD; Elena Bekker, MD; Marcelo F.K. Benveniste, MD; Sonia L. Betancourt-Cuellar, MD; David M. Biko, MD; Patrick P. Bourgouin, MD, FRCPC; Brett W. Carter, MD; Regina Chavous-Gibson, MSN, RN; Adam R. Dulberger, MD, Capt, USAF, MC; Dane A. Fisher, MD, Capt, USAF; Sherief H. Garrana, MD; Orly Goitein, MD; Allen P. Heeger, DO; Wayne L. Hofstetter, MD; Soheil Kooraki, MD; Pradeep Kuttysankaran; John P. Lichtenberger III, MD; Rachna Madan, MD; Maria A. Manning, MD; Edith M. Marom, MD; Diana P. Palacio, MD; Regina F. Parker, MA/MBA; Michael A. Pavio, MD; P. Gabriel Peterson, MD, LTC, USA; Melissa L. Rosado-de-Christenson, MD, FACR; Chad D. Strange, MD; Mylene T. Truong, MD; John Vassallo; Merissa N. Zeman, MD.

## UNAPPROVED/OFF-LABEL USE DISCLOSURE

The EOCME requires CME faculty to disclose to the participants:
1. When products or procedures being discussed are off-label, unlabelled, experimental, and/or investigational (not US Food and Drug Administration [FDA] approved); and
2. Any limitations on the information presented, such as data that are preliminary or that represent ongoing research, interim analyses, and/or unsupported opinions. Faculty may discuss information about pharmaceutical agents that is outside of FDA-approved labelling. This information is intended solely for CME and is not intended to promote off-label use of these medications. If you have any questions, contact the medical affairs department of the manufacturer for the most recent prescribing information.

## TO ENROLL

To enroll in the *Radiologic Clinics of North America* Continuing Medical Education program, call customer service at 1-800-654-2452 or sign up online at http://www.theclinics.com/home/cme. The CME program is available to subscribers for an additional annual fee of USD 356.00.

## METHOD OF PARTICIPATION

In order to claim credit, participants must complete the following:
1. Complete enrolment as indicated above.
2. Read the activity.
3. Complete the CME Test and Evaluation. Participants must achieve a score of 70% on the test. All CME Tests and Evaluations must be completed online.

## CME INQUIRIES/SPECIAL NEEDS

For all CME inquiries or special needs, please contact elsevierCME@elsevier.com.

# RADIOLOGIC CLINICS OF NORTH AMERICA

**FORTHCOMING ISSUES**

*May 2021*
**Advanced Neuroimaging in Brain Tumors**
Sangam Kanekar, *Editor*

*July 2021*
**Update on Incidental Cross-sectional Imaging Findings**
Douglas S. Katz and John J. Hines, *Editors*

*September 2021*
**PET Imaging**
Jonathan McConathy and Samuel J. Galgano, *Editors*

**RECENT ISSUES**

*January 2021*
**Breast Imaging**
Phoebe E. Freer, *Editor*

*November 2020*
**Endocrine Imaging**
Mark E. Lockhart, *Editor*

*September 2020*
**Renal Imaging**
Steven C. Eberhardt and Steven S. Raman, *Editors*

---

**RELATED SERIES**

*Advances in Clinical Radiology*
www.advancesinclinicalradiology.com
*MRI Clinics*
www.mri.theclinics.com
*Neuroimaging Clinics*
www.neuroimaging.theclinics.com
*PET Clinics*
www.pet.theclinics.com

---

**THE CLINICS ARE AVAILABLE ONLINE!**
Access your subscription at:
www.theclinics.com

# Preface
# Modern Imaging of the Mediastinum

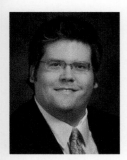

Brett W. Carter, MD
*Editor*

The mediastinum is an anatomically complex region of the thorax that includes numerous organs and structures from which a wide variety of abnormalities arise that may be of neoplastic, infectious/inflammatory, congenital, vascular, or lymphatic etiology. Scientific knowledge regarding the mediastinum and many of its associated neoplasms has advanced tremendously through the work of the International Thymic Malignancy Interest Group (ITMIG), a multidisciplinary society of experts in surgery, oncology, pathology, radiology, and neurology founded in 2010. ITMIG has developed and published numerous standards and policy papers and collaborated with the International Association for the Study of Lung Cancer to create the first standardized TNM staging system for thymic epithelial neoplasms. One of these standards is a classification system that divides the mediastinum into 3 unique compartments based on cross-sectional imaging techniques, such as computed tomography (CT), magnetic resonance (MR) imaging, and PET/CT: the prevascular, visceral, and paravertebral compartments. This modern model of the mediastinum represents a significant step forward, as cross-sectional imaging modalities are the primary method of evaluating normal structures, anatomic variants, and abnormalities in this region of the thorax. It is anticipated that the widespread implementation of this model will improve lesion characterization, assist health care professionals in generating a focused differential diagnosis for detected masses, and facilitate appropriate biopsy and treatment plans.

In this issue of the *Radiologic Clinics*, titled "Imaging of the Mediastinum," my colleagues and I present an updated exploration of the role of radiologists in the evaluation of suspected or known mediastinal disease. The articles in this issue include a wide range of topics, some of which are broad and review advances in the imaging of specific mediastinal compartments, using the ITMIG model as substrate. Others are more specific and delve into the details of the TNM staging system for such cancers as esophageal cancer and thymic epithelial neoplasms. Several radiologic-pathologic correlation articles bridge the gap between imaging findings, staging systems, and histopathologic analysis. Finally, excellent focused reviews are included on the expanding role of MR imaging in the evaluation of mediastinal abnormalities, potential pitfalls in evaluating mediastinal masses, and the methods used by interventional radiologists to biopsy and treat mediastinal lesions. I sincerely thank the authors for contributing their time and expertise to this innovative issue on imaging of the mediastinum.

Brett W. Carter, MD
Department of Thoracic Imaging
MD Anderson Cancer Center
1515 Holcombe Boulevard, Unit 1478
Houston, TX 77030, USA

*E-mail address:*
bcarter2@mdanderson.org

radiologic.theclinics.com

# International Thymic Malignancy Interest Group Model of Mediastinal Compartments

Brett W. Carter, MD

## KEYWORDS

• Mediastinum • Compartments • CT • Chest • ITMIG

## KEY POINTS

- The classification of mediastinal compartments developed by the International Thymic Malignancy Interest Group (ITMIG) has been designed for use with cross-sectional imaging examinations and is considered a standard.
- The ITMIG model divides the mediastinum into 3 unique compartments: the prevascular compartment, visceral compartment, and paravertebral compartment.
- Abnormalities originating from the prevascular compartment tend to be thymic abnormalities, germ cell neoplasms, lymphoma, metastatic disease involving lymph nodes, and goiter.
- Lesions arising in the visceral compartment include lymphadenopathy due to primary lymphoma or metastatic disease, foregut duplication cysts, tracheal lesions, esophageal neoplasms and vascular lesions originating from the heart, pericardium, and great vessels.
- Most abnormalities originating from the paravertebral compartment are neurogenic neoplasms, infections (discitis/osteomyelitis), or those related to trauma.

## INTRODUCTION

Division of the mediastinum, a region of the thorax that contains many important vascular and nonvascular organs and other anatomic structures, into specific compartments on imaging examinations has been performed for many years by clinical radiologists. Experience has shown that this exercise is extremely valuable when identifying and characterizing masses and other mediastinal abnormalities, and for ultimately determining the next step in clinical management. Several classification schemes have been created not only by radiologists but anatomists and surgeons, although their use has not been uniform. The Shields scheme has been the model most frequently used in clinical practice, whereas the Fraser and Paré's, Felson, Heitzman, Zylak, and Whitten models have been used by radiologists in clinical practice.[1–7]

The limitations of existing classification schemes have been well-documented and include significant variations in the terminology and methods used for the identification of individual compartments, which has resulted in miscommunication between health care professionals and the inability to reliably localize some lesions to a specific compartment, and, on the imaging side, the use of arbitrary nonanatomic divisions of the thorax that are based principally on the lateral chest radiograph. In response to the need for a model of the mediastinal compartments designed for use with cross-sectional imaging techniques

Department of Thoracic Imaging, MD Anderson Cancer Center, 1515 Holcombe Boulevard, Unit 1478, Houston, TX 77030, USA
E-mail address: bcarter2@mdanderson.org

Radiol Clin N Am 59 (2021) 149–153
https://doi.org/10.1016/j.rcl.2020.11.007
0033-8389/21/© 2020 Elsevier Inc. All rights reserved.

such as computed tomography (CT), MR imaging, and PET/CT, which are the imaging modalities primarily used in the identification and characterization of mediastinal masses, a new, modern classification scheme has been developed by the International Thymic Malignancy Interest Group (ITMIG), building on prior work by the Japanese Association for Research on the Thymus (JART).[8] In this article, the ITMIG model is illustrated with representative examples.

## INTERNATIONAL THYMIC MALIGNANCY INTEREST GROUP MODEL DEFINITIONS

The rationale for and methodology used by ITMIG in the development of this classification scheme has been previously described.[9,10] The model developed by ITMIG includes 3 unique compartments: the prevascular compartment (corresponding to the anterior compartment on chest radiography), the visceral compartment (corresponding to the middle compartment on chest radiography), and the paravertebral compartment (corresponding to the posterior compartment on chest radiography) (Table 1). The specific boundaries of each department and the anatomic organs and structures that they normally contain can be easily identified on cross-sectional imaging examinations (Fig. 1). Understanding this model enables the radiologist to predict what lesions are most likely to originate from specific mediastinal compartments.

### Prevascular Mediastinal Compartment

The prevascular mediastinal compartment has the following boundaries: (1) superiorly, the thoracic inlet, (2) inferiorly, the diaphragm, (3) anteriorly, the posterior border/cortex of the sternum, (4) laterally, the parietal mediastinal pleura, and (5) posteriorly, the anterior aspect of the pericardium. Using these anatomic landmarks, the most significant organs and structures contained in the prevascular compartment include the thymus, fat, lymph nodes, and the left brachiocephalic vein. The most common lesions to arise from the prevascular compartment are thymic abnormalities (cysts, hyperplasia, and thymic epithelial neoplasms including thymoma, thymic carcinoma, and neuroendocrine tumors), germ cell neoplasms, lymphoma, metastatic disease involving lymph nodes, and goiter (Fig. 2).

### Visceral Mediastinal Compartment

The visceral mediastinal compartment has the following boundaries: (1) superiorly, the thoracic inlet, (2) inferiorly, the diaphragm, (3) anteriorly, the posterior boundaries of the prevascular

**Table 1**
**ITMIG classification of mediastinal compartments**

| Compartment | Boundaries | Contents |
|---|---|---|
| Prevascular | Superior: thoracic inlet<br>Inferior: diaphragm<br>Anterior: sternum<br>Lateral: parietal mediastinal pleura<br>Posterior: anterior aspect of the pericardium as it wraps around the heart in a curvilinear fashion | Thymus<br>Fat<br>Lymph nodes<br>Left brachiocephalic vein |
| Visceral | Superior: thoracic inlet<br>Inferior: diaphragm<br>Anterior: posterior boundaries of the prevascular compartment<br>Posterior: vertical line connecting a point on each thoracic vertebral body 1 cm posterior to its anterior margin | Nonvascular: trachea, carina, esophagus, lymph nodes<br>Vascular: heart, ascending thoracic aorta, aortic arch, descending thoracic aorta, superior vena cava, intrapericardial pulmonary arteries, thoracic duct |
| Paravertebral | Superior: thoracic inlet<br>Inferior: diaphragm<br>Anterior: posterior boundaries of the visceral compartment<br>Posterolateral: vertical line against the posterior margin of the chest wall at the lateral margin of the transverse process of the thoracic spine | Thoracic spine<br>Paravertebral soft tissues |

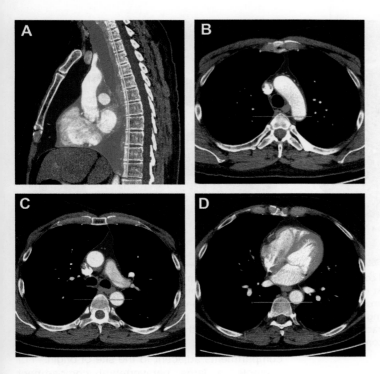

Fig. 1. ITMIG Definition of Mediastinal Compartments. Sagittal reformatted CT image (*A*) and axial CT images at the levels of the aortic arch (*B*), left pulmonary artery (*C*), and left atrium (*D*) demonstrate the model developed by ITMIG. The prevascular compartment (*blue*) wraps around the heart and pericardium, which are located in the visceral compartment (*red*). Purple = paravertebral compartment; yellow line = visceral-paravertebral compartment boundary line.

compartment, and (4) posteriorly, a vertical line connecting a point on the thoracic vertebral bodies 1 cm posterior to the anterior margin of the spine, referred to as the visceral–paravertebral compartment boundary line (see Table 1). Using these anatomic landmarks, the most significant organs and structures contained in the visceral compartment may be either vascular (the heart, superior vena cava, ascending thoracic aorta, aortic arch, descending thoracic aorta, intrapericardial pulmonary arteries, and thoracic duct) or nonvascular (the trachea, carina, esophagus, and lymph nodes). Of note, all structures within the pericardium are localized to the visceral compartment in the ITMIG classification system. The most common abnormalities in the visceral compartment include lymphadenopathy due to primary lymphoma or metastatic disease, foregut duplication cysts (bronchogenic and esophageal duplication cysts), tracheal lesions, esophageal neoplasms and vascular lesions originating from the heart, pericardium, and great vessels (**Fig. 3**).

## Paravertebral Mediastinal Compartment

The paravertebral mediastinal compartment has the following boundaries: (1) superiorly, the thoracic inlet, (2) inferiorly, the diaphragm, (3) anteriorly, the posterior boundaries of the visceral compartment, and (4) posterolaterally, a vertical line along the posterior margin of the chest wall at the lateral aspect of the transverse processes (see **Table 1**). Using these anatomic landmarks, the most significant organs and structures

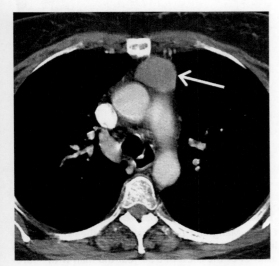

Fig. 2. Thymoma in the prevascular compartment. Contrast-enhanced axial CT of the chest of a 64-year-old woman with myasthenia gravis demonstrates a focal soft tissue mass (*arrow*) in the prevascular compartment consistent with a biopsy-proven thymoma.

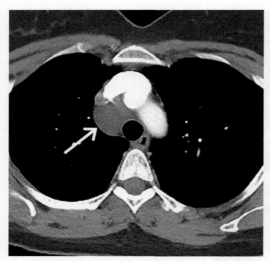

**Fig. 3.** Bronchogenic cyst in the visceral compartment. Contrast-enhanced axial CT of the chest of a 50-year-old woman demonstrates a well-circumscribed, fluid attenuation lesion (*arrow*), representing a broncho-genic cyst, located in the right paratracheal region, confirming its location in the visceral compartment.

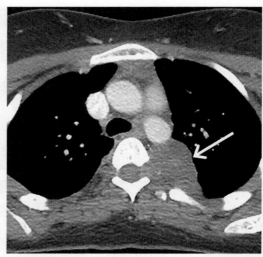

**Fig. 4.** Schwannoma in the paravertebral compart-ment. Contrast-enhanced axial CT of the chest of a 27-year-old woman shows a heterogeneous mass (*ar-row*) in the left paraspinal region, localizing this neurofibroma to the paravertebral compartment.

contained in the paravertebral compartment include the thoracic spine and paravertebral soft tissues. The most common lesions originating from the paravertebral compartment are neuro-genic neoplasms, infections (discitis/osteomye-litis), or those related to trauma (hematoma), although a wide variety of miscellaneous lesions related to other underlying conditions (such as extramedullary hematopoiesis) are possible (**Fig. 4**).

## LOCALIZATION CONSIDERATIONS

Although most normal organs and anatomic struc-tures, variants, and associated abnormalities can typically be localized to an individual compartment using the ITMIG model, accomplishing this goal may be difficult depending on several factors. One of the most common scenarios is a large mediastinal mass that involves multiple compart-ments. ITMIG has described 2 tools—the center method and the structure displacement tool—that can assist the radiologist in identifying the compartment of origin. The center method, which was also used in the JART study, stipulates that the center point of a lesion, as visualized on the axial image showing its greatest size, can deter-mine the compartment of origin[8] (**Fig. 5**). The structure displacement tool can be used when large mediastinal abnormalities displace organs and anatomic structures in other mediastinal

compartments adjacent to the site of origin.[9] For example, a large paravertebral compartment mass may anteriorly displace organs of the visceral mediastinal compartment, such as the heart.

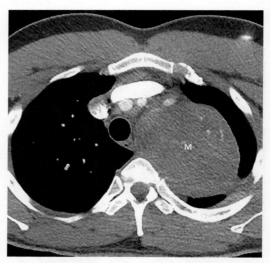

**Fig. 5.** Malignant peripheral nerve sheath neoplasm involving multiple compartments. Contrast-enhanced axial CT of the chest of a 30-year-old man with neuro-fibromatosis type 1 demonstrates a large mass (*M*) in the left mediastinum. Using the center method, the mass is centered in the left paravertebral compart-ment but extends to also involve the visceral medias-tinal compartment. CT-guided biopsy revealed malignant peripheral nerve sheath tumor.

## SUMMARY

The ITMIG definition of mediastinal compartments is a modern classification scheme developed using cross-sectional imaging techniques that has been accepted as a standard. As imaging modalities such as CT, MR imaging, and PET/CT are the primary methods of evaluating mediastinal abnormalities, using this model will improve lesion characterization, assist health care professionals in generating a focused differential diagnosis for detected masses, and facilitate appropriate biopsy and treatment plans.

## DISCLOSURE

Nothing to disclose for all authors.

## REFERENCES

1. Shields TW. Primary tumors and cysts of the mediastinum. In: Shields TW, editor. General thoracic surgery. Philadelphia: Lea & Febiger; 1983. p. 927–54.

2. The mediastinum. In: Fraser RS, Müller NL, Colman N, et al, editors. Fraser and Paré's diagnosis of diseases of the chest. 4th edition. Philadelphia: Saunders; 1999. p. 196–234.

3. The normal chest. In: Fraser RG, Paré PA, editors. Diagnosis of diseases of the chest. 2nd edition. Philadelphia: Saunders; 1977. p. 1–183.

4. Felson B. Chest roentgenology. Philadelphia: Saunders; 1973.

5. Heitzman ER. The mediastinum. 2nd edition. New York: Springer-Verlag; 1988.

6. Zylak CJ, Pallie W, Jackson R. Correlative anatomy and computed tomography: a module on the mediastinum. Radiographics 1982;2(4):555–92.

7. Whitten CR, Khan S, Munneke GJ, et al. A diagnostic approach to mediastinal abnormalities. Radiographics 2007;27(3):657–71.

8. Fujimoto K, Hara M, Tomiyama N, et al. Proposal for a new mediastinal compartment classification of transverse plane images according to the Japanese Association for Research on the Thymus (JART) general rules for the study of mediastinal tumors. Oncol Rep 2014;31(2):565–72.

9. Carter BW, Tomiyama N, Bhora FY, et al. A modern definition of mediastinal compartments. J Thorac Oncol 2014;9(9 suppl 2):S97–101.

10. Carter BW, Benveniste MF, Madan R, et al. ITMIG classification of mediastinal compartments and multidisciplinary approach to mediastinal masses. Radiographics 2017;37(2):413–36.

# Imaging of the Anterior/Prevascular Mediastinum

Sherief H. Garrana, MD[a,b,*], Melissa L. Rosado-de-Christenson, MD[a,b]

## KEYWORDS

- Prevascular mediastinum • Thymic hyperplasia • Thymic cyst • Thymic epithelial neoplasm
- Thymoma • Thymic carcinoid • Germ cell neoplasm

## KEY POINTS

- Various neoplastic and non-neoplastic entities may affect the prevascular mediastinum.
- Most prevascular mediastinal masses are discovered incidentally and are characterized further with contrast-enhanced chest computed tomography.
- Correlation of specific imaging features with demographic and clinical information may allow radiologists to provide a focused differential or a specific diagnosis.
- By distinguishing surgical from nonsurgical lesions, radiologists play a crucial role in the multidisciplinary approach to the management of prevascular mediastinal pathologies.

## INTRODUCTION

The mediastinum contains many organs, structures, and tissues. A wide variety of entities may arise primarily from these structures or secondarily involve this region, including neoplasms, glandular enlargement, congenital and vascular abnormalities, lymphadenopathy, and mesenchymal lesions. Localization of mediastinal masses to specific compartments, together with demographic and clinical information, allows formulation of a focused differential diagnosis and helps guide further evaluation and management. Anterior, middle, and posterior mediastinal compartments have been used for decades in radiographic interpretation.[1] The International Thymic Malignancy Interest Group recently redefined the mediastinal compartments based on cross-sectional imaging, separating the mediastinum into prevascular, visceral, and paravertebral compartments. Contents of the prevascular compartment include the thymus, fat, lymph nodes, left brachiocephalic vein, small vessels, nerves, and lymphatic channels. The most common pathologies that occur in this compartment include thymic lesions, germ cell neoplasms

(GCNs), lymphoma, lymphatic malformations, metastatic disease, and glandular lesions.[2]

Mediastinal masses are uncommon. They typically are discovered on radiography and are characterized further with computed tomography (CT) and/or MR imaging. More than half of all mediastinal masses arise from the prevascular compartment.[3] When classic imaging features are present, a specific diagnosis may be suggested based solely on CT imaging features. The appearances of prevascular mediastinal lesions may overlap, however, and additional imaging studies, laboratory tests, and tissue sampling often are required for a definitive diagnosis.

The true incidence of prevascular mediastinal masses is difficult to determine largely due to historical variability in clinical and radiologic classification systems of mediastinal compartments in published studies, which may or may not include congenital and nonsurgical lesions and due to variability regarding the inclusion of lymphoma.[4] The most common tumors of the prevascular mediastinum are thymic epithelial neoplasms and lymphoma. Other neoplasms include neuroendocrine tumors, GCNs, and a variety of thymic neoplasms. The most common non-neoplastic masses are

a Department of Radiology, Saint Luke's Hospital of Kansas City, 4401 Wornall Road, Kansas City, MO 64111, USA; b University of Missouri-Kansas City School of Medicine, 2411 Holmes Street, Kansas City, MO 64108, USA
* Corresponding author. Department of Radiology, Saint Luke's Hospital of Kansas City, 4401 Wornall Road, Kansas City, MO 64111.
E-mail address: Sherief.garrana@gmail.com

Radiol Clin N Am 59 (2021) 155–168
https://doi.org/10.1016/j.rcl.2020.10.003
0033-8389/21/© 2020 Elsevier Inc. All rights reserved.

cystic lesions, which may be congenital or acquired. Vascular abnormalities, lymphatic malformations, mediastinal thyroid and parathyroid tissue, and thymic enlargement also may occur.

## IMAGING OF THE PREVASCULAR MEDIASTINUM
### Radiography

Chest radiography is the imaging study performed most commonly and often is the first imaging modality to demonstrate a mediastinal abnormality. A systematic approach to radiographic analysis and knowledge of normal mediastinal lines, stripes, and interfaces allow radiologists to identify and localize mediastinal lesions. Although small mediastinal lesions may produce normal or subtle findings, large lesions typically produce contour abnormalities or distortion of the aforementioned lines, stripes, and interfaces on posteroanterior (PA) radiography (**Fig. 1**). The lateral radiograph then is used to localize the lesion to the anterior mediastinum. Identification of the hilum overlay sign allows differentiation of an anterior mediastinal lesion from a hilar mass.[1]

### Computed Tomography

Contrast-enhanced CT is the modality of choice for evaluating mediastinal masses and is equal to or superior to MR imaging in diagnosing most lesions, with the exception of thymic cysts.[5] CT analysis of a prevascular mediastinal lesion should be systematic and should address multiple characteristics, including (1) location, size, morphology, and margins; (2) density/attenuation and enhancement characteristics;

(3) internal composition, including soft tissue, fat, fluid, and calcification; (4) relationship with adjacent structures, including mass effect and/or invasion; and (5) presence or absence of lymphadenopathy.[4]

### MR Imaging

MR imaging is not performed routinely for the assessment of mediastinal masses but is the optimal imaging modality for distinguishing cystic from solid lesions, identifying cystic and/or necrotic lesion components, characterizing cystic lesions as to the presence of septations and mural nodularity, and distinguishing normal or hyperplastic thymic tissue from neoplasia.[6]

### Fluorodeoxyglucose PET/Computed Tomography

[18]F-fluorodeoxyglucose (FDG) PET/CT has a limited role in the evaluation of mediastinal masses and often is nonspecific given that many infectious and inflammatory processes result in increased FDG uptake, which can be mistaken for malignancy. Although FDG PET/CT has been used to distinguish between low-grade thymoma, high-grade thymoma, and thymic carcinoma,[7,8] there is significant overlap between FDG-avid neoplasms, including high-grade thymic epithelial neoplasms, lymphoma, paraganglioma, and nonseminomatous malignant GCNs.[9] FDG PET/CT, however, is the imaging modality of choice for staging and restaging lymphoma. The overall consensus suggests that FDG PET/CT may have an ancillary role in the diagnostic workup of prevascular mediastinal masses, but accuracy and

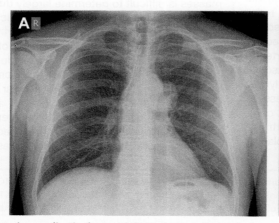
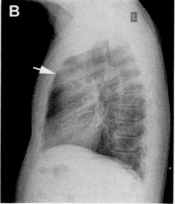

Fig. 1. Anterior mediastinal mass. (*A*) PA chest radiograph shows a left mediastinal mass that demonstrates the hilum overlay sign. (*B*) Lateral chest radiograph allows localization of the mass to the anterior mediastinum (*arrow*). Thymoma subsequently was diagnosed.

specificity are limited, with significant overlap between different mediastinal pathologies.[9–11]

## THYMIC HYPERPLASIA

Normal thymic tissue typically is identified in the prevascular mediastinum of young patients and gradually decreases with age, with fatty replacement usually complete by age 40. When uniform thymic enlargement with a bilobed morphology and intercalated fat is present, thymic hyperplasia is the leading consideration. Rebound hyperplasia is defined as an increase in thymic volume by greater than 50% compared with baseline and typically occurs after chemotherapy, radiation therapy, prolonged corticosteroid treatment, or after physiologic stress from severe injuries or burns. Thymic hyperplasia, specifically lymphoid (follicular) hyperplasia, is characterized by thymic lymphoid follicles with or without concurrent increase in glandular size. It typically occurs in patients with underlying systemic disorders, such as myasthenia gravis, collagen vascular disease, systemic lupus erythematosus, human immunodeficiency virus infection, and hyperthyroidism[12] (Fig. 2A).

Thymic hyperplasia may manifest on CT as a diffuse, focal, or asymmetric nodular or masslike heterogeneous soft tissue lesion with lobular margins and may mimic a mediastinal neoplasm. If suspicion for thymic hyperplasia is high, short-term interval follow-up CT can be obtained, with an expected decrease in size. Alternatively, chemical-shift MR imaging may be performed to confirm intralesional fat, an expected finding in thymic hyperplasia (Fig. 2B), or suggest the diagnosis of thymic neoplasia.[13]

## THYMIC EPITHELIAL NEOPLASMS

Thymic epithelial neoplasms are rare and account for 0.2% to 1.5% of all malignancies in the United States, but are the most common nonlymphomatous primary neoplasm of the prevascular mediastinum.[14,15] These tumors include thymomas and thymic carcinomas. Complete resection when possible is the treatment of choice for these neoplasms. Neoadjuvant and/or adjuvant systemic therapy and radiation often are utilized for invasive lesions.[16,17]

### Thymoma

Thymoma is the most common primary neoplasm of the prevascular mediastinum and is the most common thymic epithelial neoplasm, with a reported 0.15 cases per 100,000 persons, accounting for 20% of prevascular mediastinal masses in adults.[18,19] The highest incidence occurs in middle-aged patients, typically between 40 years and 60 years, without gender predilection.[12,20] These generally are slow-growing encapsulated neoplasms but may invade vascular structures and/or involve the pleura and pericardium. Distant metastases are rare.[14,21] Affected patients may be asymptomatic, may have symptoms related to mass effect or local invasion, or may present with a paraneoplastic syndrome. Such parathymic syndromes include myasthenia gravis, pure red cell aplasia/Diamond-Blackfan syndrome, aplastic

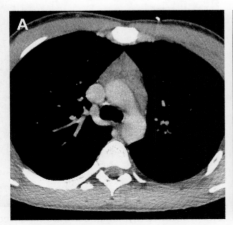
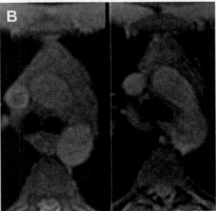

Fig. 2. Thymic hyperplasia secondary to Graves disease. (*A*) Contrast-enhanced axial CT shows diffuse thymic enlargement with soft tissue attenuation and intercalated fat. (*B*) Composite image of chemical-shift MR imaging shows in-phase homogeneous high signal intensity in the thymus (*left*) and signal drop on out-of-phase imaging (*right*), consistent with thymic hyperplasia. Follicular hyperplasia was suspected, given associated hyperthyroidism.

anemia, and hypogammaglobulinemia. Thymomas are also associated with autoimmune disorders such as Hashimoto's thyroiditis, systemic lupus erythematosus, polymyositis, and rheumatoid arthritis.[22–24] The most common symptoms reported at presentation are chest pain, dyspnea, cough, dysphagia, diaphragmatic paralysis, and superior vena cava (SVC) syndrome.

More than 80% of thymomas are diagnosed accurately on CT or MR imaging.[5] CT of suspected thymoma should be performed with contrast for more accurate identification of invasive features. Thymoma should be the leading diagnostic consideration when a homogeneous or slightly heterogeneous rounded or lobular prevascular mediastinal mass is present in a patient over the age of 40. A tissue plane between the mass and adjacent structures may be visible in encapsulated lesions (**Fig. 3**). Heterogeneity within the mass due to internal cystic or necrotic foci, irregular lobular contours, and intrinsic calcifications suggest invasive thymoma[25,26] (**Figs. 4** and **5**). Invasive lesions may exhibit infiltration of the mediastinal fat, vascular encasement or frank invasion, and/or pleural and pericardial metastases. Lymphadenopathy typically is absent. The presence of local invasion, lymphadenopathy, pleural effusion, or distant metastases should raise concern for more aggressive neoplasms, such as thymic carcinoma or carcinoid (**Fig. 6**).

## *Thymic Carcinoma*

Thymic carcinomas are uncommon but represent approximately 20% of thymic epithelial neoplasms, and affected patients are often symptomatic. The mean age at presentation is 50 years.[14] Imaging features may be indistinguishable from those of thymoma, but thymic carcinoma typically exhibits aggressive features, such as invasion of adjacent structures, lymphadenopathy, pleural/pericardial effusions, and distant metastases (**Fig. 7**). Approximately 50% to 65% of patients have distant metastases at the time of diagnosis.[14] In contrast to thymoma, paraneoplastic syndromes rarely are associated with thymic carcinoma.

## THYMIC NEUROENDOCRINE NEOPLASMS

Thymic neuroendocrine neoplasms are the least common primary thymic tumors, comprising 2% to 5% of these lesions, and most frequently are carcinoids, specifically atypical carcinoids.[27] The reported median age at presentation is 57 years, with a 3:1 male-to-female ratio.[28] Approximately 25% develop in patients with multiple endocrine neoplasia (MEN) type 1.[29] Most patients are symptomatic at diagnosis secondary to local invasion and mass effect and may present with paraneoplastic syndromes, most commonly Cushing syndrome, due to ectopic production of

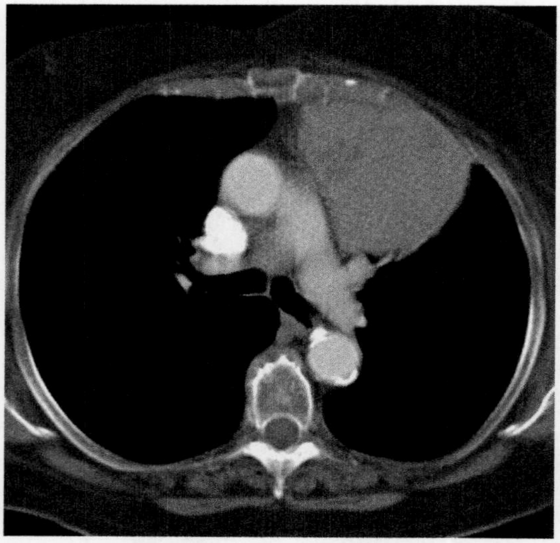

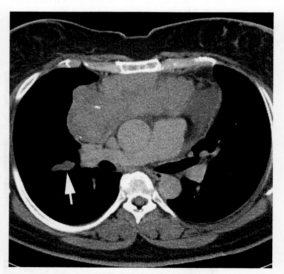

**Fig. 3.** Thymoma. Contrast-enhanced axial CT shows an enhancing left prevascular mass with a distinct tissue plane separating the mass from the adjacent pulmonary trunk. Surgical excision showed a thymoma with microscopic invasion of the adjacent mediastinal fat.

**Fig. 4.** Invasive thymoma. Contrast-enhanced axial CT shows a large, lobulated, heterogeneously enhancing, prevascular mediastinal mass with intrinsic calcification and absence of a tissue plane between it and the pericardium, concerning for invasion. Note right pleural metastasis along the major fissure (*arrow*).

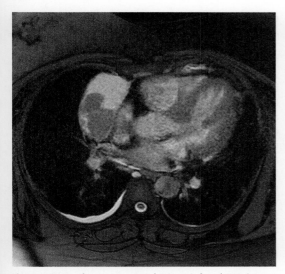

Fig. 5. Cystic thymoma. Axial T2-weighted MR image with fat suppression shows a large, right prevascular mediastinal cystic mass with T2 hyperintense signal corresponding to fluid in the lesion as well as eccentric soft tissue nodules.

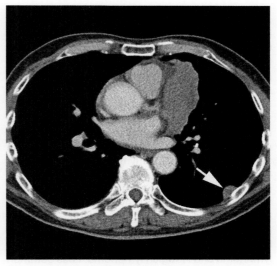

Fig. 6. Invasive thymoma. Contrast-enhanced axial CT shows a heterogeneously enhancing left prevascular mediastinal mass with pericardial invasion and a left pleural metastasis (*arrow*).

adrenocorticotropic hormone. Other paraneoplastic syndrome of inappropriate secretion of antidiuretic hormone (SIADH), and rarely carcinoid syndrome.[14] Approximately one-third of affected patients are asymptomatic and may be diagnosed incidentally or during surveillance for MEN 1.[27]

On imaging, these typically are aggressive, prevascular mediastinal soft tissue masses that may invade surrounding structures and often are associated with mediastinal lymphadenopathy[30] (Fig. 8). Surgical resection is the treatment of choice, with or without adjuvant or neoadjuvant systemic therapy and/or radiation therapy.

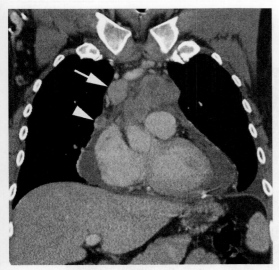

Fig. 7. Thymic carcinoma. Contrast-enhanced coronal CT shows a heterogeneously enhancing, necrotic prevascular mediastinal mass with lymphadenopathy (*arrow*), solid pericardial metastasis (*arrowhead*), and a pericardial effusion.

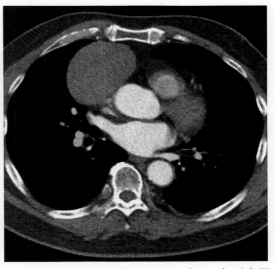

Fig. 8. Thymic carcinoid. Contrast-enhanced axial CT demonstrates a homogenous right prevascular mediastinal mass abutting the pericardium. Atypical carcinoid tumor was confirmed after surgery.

## LYMPHOMA

Lymphomas are heterogeneous neoplasms with frequent intrathoracic involvement and account for 4.9% of newly diagnosed malignancies. Lymphoma may arise primarily in the mediastinum or secondarily may involve it. A diagnosis of lymphoma should be favored over thymoma in younger patients and in those with a mediastinal mass and associated lymphadenopathy. Primary mediastinal lymphomas are rare, comprising approximately 1% of all lymphomas.[31] Diagnosis of primary mediastinal lymphoma necessitates involvement of mediastinal lymph nodes, the thymus, or both, without evidence of extranodal or systemic disease at presentation. The most common cell types to primarily or secondarily involve the mediastinum are diffuse large B-cell lymphoma and Hodgkin lymphoma. Less common cell types include primary mediastinal (thymic) B-cell lymphoma, gray zone lymphoma (GZL), T-cell lymphoblastic lymphoma (TCLL), mucosa-associated lymphoid tissue (MALT) lymphoma, and peripheral T-cell lymphoma (PTCL).[31,32]

Lymphoma should be considered when large, lobular, soft tissue masses and/or enlarged lymph nodes are identified in the prevascular mediastinum, particularly if there is involvement of other mediastinal compartments and lymph node stations or infiltration between or encasement of vascular structures, with or without mass effect or local invasion (Fig. 9A). Systemic B symptoms, such as fever, night sweats, and weight loss, in combination with typical imaging features, are highly suggestive of the diagnosis. More aggressive subtypes, such as GZL and TCLL, often exhibit increased heterogeneity and invasion of adjacent structures.[31]

FDG PET/CT is the imaging modality of choice for initial staging and ongoing surveillance of patients with lymphoma. Studies have shown increased accuracy of FDG PET/CT in detecting lymph node involvement and identifying intranodal and extranodal disease throughout the body as compared with CT. FDG PET/CT may identify occult lesions in the spleen, gastrointestinal tract, and bones. FDG PET/CT also can be used to guide tissue sampling, with the goal of sampling the most FDG-avid foci and avoid necrotic or uninvolved tissue (Fig. 9B). Low-grade lymphomas, such as MALT lymphoma and PTCL, often demonstrate minimal to no FDG uptake on PET/CT.[33]

## GERM CELL NEOPLASMS

GCNs are a heterogenous group of tumors that comprise 10% to 15% of adult prevascular mediastinal masses and are thought to originate from primitive germ cells aberrantly placed in the mediastinum during embryogenesis. The prevascular mediastinum is the most common extragonadal site for these tumors, which are histologically identical to their gonadal counterparts, and encompass teratomas, seminomas, and nonseminomatous malignant GCNs. GCNs may mimic other prevascular mediastinal masses, and demographic information, clinical history, and serology often help suggest the correct diagnosis.

### Teratoma

Teratomas are the most common mediastinal GCNs and are composed of tissues derived from

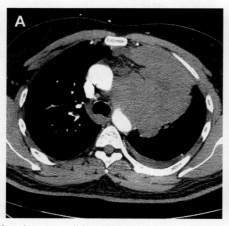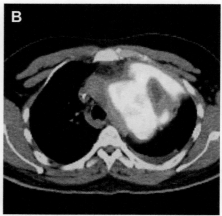

**Fig. 9.** Diffuse large B-cell lymphoma. (*A*) Contrast-enhanced axial CT shows a heterogeneously enhancing mass involving the left prevascular mediastinum extending into the visceral compartment and compressing and/or invading adjacent vessels and the left lung. (*B*) Fused axial FDG PET/CT shows extensive FDG avidity in the mass with low uptake foci representing necrosis.

more than 1 of the 3 primitive germ cell layers. These tumors can contain ectodermal (teeth, skin, and hair), mesodermal (cartilage and bone), and endodermal derivatives (bronchial, intestinal, and pancreatic tissue). A vast majority are mature teratomas and are histologically well differentiated and benign. Immature teratomas are rare variants that contain fetal tissue, are considered malignant, and carry a good prognosis when diagnosed in children but may recur locally or metastasize in adults. Rarely, teratomas may contain intrinsic foci of carcinoma, sarcoma, or malignant GCN, in which case they are referred to as *malignant teratoma* or *teratocarcinoma*.[34]

Mature teratomas represent 60% to 70% of mediastinal GCNs and typically affect children and young adults without gender predilection. Affected patients often are asymptomatic. Symptoms, when present, usually are due to large lesions that produce mass effect and compression of surrounding structures and include chest pain, dyspnea, cough, and dysphagia. If the tumors contain ectopic intestinal mucosal or exocrine pancreatic tissue, secreted enzymes may result in rupture into the tracheobronchial tree, pleura, pericardium, or lung. Expectoration of hair (trichoptysis) or sebum is rare but pathognomonic for ruptured mediastinal teratoma.[34,35]

On cross-sectional imaging, these tumors are unilateral well-defined encapsulated lesions with rounded or lobular margins and intrinsic heterogeneity, including cystic foci and solid components, that may include soft tissue and calcification. Many mature teratomas exhibit predominantly or entirely unilocular or multilocular thin-walled cystic morphology, with internal septations of variable thickness and contrast enhancement, in which case they may be referred to as *cystic teratomas*. Fat occurs in 75% of lesions and may be adipose tissue or lipid within a cystic component. Rarely, intrinsic bone or teeth may be visible on imaging. A combination of fluid, soft tissue, calcium, and/or fat attenuation in a well-defined prevascular mediastinal mass is highly specific for mature teratoma (**Fig. 10**). Intrinsic fat-fluid levels are rare but diagnostic findings. Surgical resection is curative.[35]

## Seminoma

Seminomas represent approximately 40% of malignant GCNs of a single histology and occur almost exclusively in young men between the ages of 20 years to 40 years. Although some patients are asymptomatic, most have symptoms related to large tumor size resulting in compression of adjacent structures.

On cross-sectional imaging, these tumors usually manifest as a large, prevascular, mediastinal homogenous or slightly heterogeneous mass with lobulated contours that may involve other compartments or exhibit associated lymphadenopathy and thus mimic lymphoma. Invasion of adjacent structures and obliteration of intervening tissue planes may occur. Calcification is exceedingly rare. Metastases to regional lymph nodes and distant sites (in particular, osseous metastases) occasionally occur[20,34] (**Fig. 11**).

Curative therapy may consist of a combination of adjuvant or neoadjuvant chemotherapy, chemoradiation, and surgical resection, with excellent long-term survival.[12,34,36]

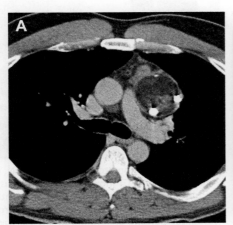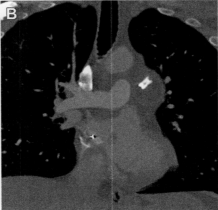

**Fig. 10.** Mature teratoma. (*A*) Contrast-enhanced axial CT shows a well-defined left prevascular mediastinal mass with intrinsic fat, soft tissue, and densely calcified/ossified components. (*B*) Contrast-enhanced coronal CT (bone window) shows a calcified structure within the mass that represented a well-formed tooth.

### Nonseminomatous Malignant Germ Cell Neoplasm

Nonseminomatous malignant germ cell neoplasms (NSGCNs) include embryonal carcinoma, yolk-sac (endodermal sinus) tumor, choriocarcinoma, mixed germ cell tumors composed of multiple histologic types, and immature and malignant teratomas. NSGCNs almost exclusively affect young adult men, with a mean age of 30 years at presentation. Affected patients have an increased risk for developing hematologic malignancies, and approximately 20% have Klinefelter syndrome.[37–39] Patients typically are symptomatic at presentation due to compression or invasion of mediastinal structures, and the severity of symptoms correlates with tumor size. On serology, elevated α-fetoprotein and β-human chorionic gonadotropin hormone levels occur in more than 50% of patients.[40] Serum lactate dehydrogenase is elevated in more than 50% of patients and tends to correlate with tumor burden rather than tumor histology.

On cross-sectional imaging, these tumors usually manifest as large, well-circumscribed or poorly-defined prevascular mediastinal masses, with extensive intrinsic heterogeneity due to necrosis, hemorrhage, and cystic change, with peripheral enhancing frondlike soft tissue.[34] These lesions frequently affect both sides of midline, with obliteration of tissue planes, and mass effect and/or invasion of adjacent structures. Pleural and pericardial metastases are common. Regional lymph node and distal metastases also occur[20,34,41–44] (Fig. 12).

NSGCNs tend to respond well to systemic chemotherapy, which usually is followed by surgical resection.[40] Serum biomarkers are helpful for ongoing disease surveillance. Affected patients have an average 5-year survival rate of 50%.[20] Patients with mediastinal NSGCNs have a poorer prognosis that those with primary gonadal tumors of the same histology.[12,36,45]

## CYSTS
### Thymic Cyst

Thymic cysts are rare, represent approximately 3% of all prevascular mediastinal masses, and may be congenital or acquired.[34,46–48] Congenital thymic cysts may be found anywhere along the embryologic course of the thymus as it descends from the neck into the prevascular mediastinum. Approximately 50% of congenital thymic cysts are discovered incidentally in the first 2 decades of life. Acquired thymic cysts usually are postinflammatory and may be associated with mediastinal malignancy, surgery, chemotherapy, radiation therapy, or trauma.[46–48]

Congenital thymic cysts typically are smaller than 6 cm, spherical, unilocular, and thin-walled. Acquired cysts may range in size from

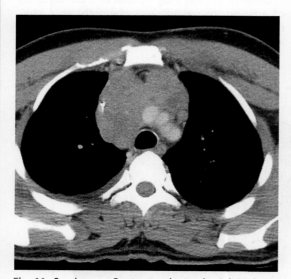

**Fig. 11.** Seminoma. Contrast-enhanced axial CT shows a locally invasive, relatively homogeneous prevascular mediastinal soft tissue mass that extends into the visceral mediastinum and obliterates the brachiocephalic veins and upper superior vena cava.

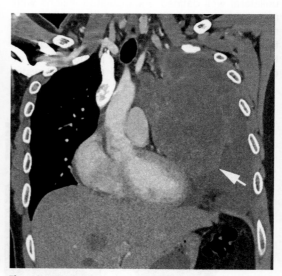

**Fig. 12.** Nonseminomatous malignant GCN. Contrast-enhanced coronal CT shows a heterogeneous, left prevascular mediastinal mass with predominantly central low attenuation corresponding to necrosis, and frondlike peripheral enhancement (*arrow*). Note mass effect on the mediastinum, left pleural effusion, and hepatic metastases. Tissue sampling confirmed yolk-sac tumor.

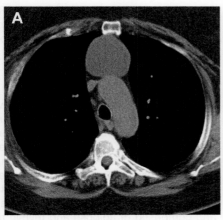
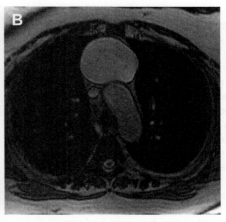

**Fig. 13.** Thymic cyst. (*A*) Unenhanced axial CT shows a large water attenuation mass in the prevascular mediastinum. (*B*) Axial T2-weighted MR image shows a thin-walled cyst with homogeneous high signal intensity throughout the lesion, consistent with a simple thymic cyst.

3 cm to 17 cm and usually are multilocular with variable wall thickness, enhancement, and/or calcification. When thymic cysts occur in the absence of symptoms and exhibit a unilocular morphology with simple fluid attenuation on CT, no further follow-up is needed (**Fig. 13**). When areas of high attenuation are present secondary to hemorrhage or proteinaceous material, internal septa, wall thickening, or mural nodularity, further characterization with MR imaging should be performed to help differentiate a complex thymic cyst from a cystic neoplasm. Surgical excision is curative in symptomatic patients or in patients in whom imaging features are equivocal.[6]

## Pericardial Cyst

Pericardial cysts are benign, non-neoplastic, congenital cysts that arise from aberrant embryologic development of the somatic or coelomic cavities. Patients typically are asymptomatic, with most cases diagnosed incidentally on imaging. Pericardial cysts typically manifest as well-circumscribed unilocular cysts of variable size and simple fluid attenuation with an imperceptible wall and are located at one of the cardiophrenic angles, more commonly the right. They may occur anywhere along the pericardium and may be located as high as the superior pericardial reflection at the aortic root and pulmonary trunk (**Fig. 14**). When imaging findings are characteristic, no imaging follow-up or treatment is needed in the absence of complications, such as superimposed infection.[45]

## LYMPHATIC AND VASCULAR LESIONS
### Mediastinal Lymphangioma

Mediastinal lymphangioma is a benign proliferation of lymphatic channels and sacs that typically occurs in very young children, with 50% present at birth and 90% discovered by 2 years of age. Rarely, lymphangiomas may manifest as primary mediastinal tumors in adults.[34]

These lesions typically occur in the superior portion of the prevascular mediastinum and usually are contiguous with cervical and/or axillary components. They may manifest as rounded,

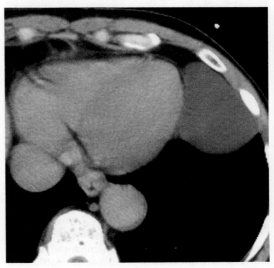

**Fig. 14.** Pericardial cyst. Contrast-enhanced axial CT shows a homogenous water attenuation cyst in the left cardiophrenic angle with an imperceptible wall.

lobulated, and multilocular cystic masses that may grow to large sizes and may infiltrate between mediastinal structures. Cystic foci correspond to dilated lymphatic channels and range from 1-2 mm in size to several centimeters. The fluid within the cystic spaces typically is of simple water attenuation, and septa may vary in thickness, sometimes with mild contrast enhancement. MR imaging is useful for further evaluating and characterizing these lesions (**Fig. 15**). Complete surgical resection often is challenging owing to their complex infiltrative nature; therefore, postsurgical surveillance often is necessary to monitor for recurrence.[34] Percutaneous sclerotherapy with injectable sclerosing agents is a potential nonsurgical treatment option for some patients.[49,50]

### Mediastinal Hemangioma

Hemangiomas are rare mediastinal tumors, which typically occur in young patients, with approximately 75% manifesting in patients under the age of 35. Up to 50% of affected patients are asymptomatic.

Mediastinal hemangiomas may occur within any mediastinal compartment and may involve more than 1 compartment, with a reported incidence of 43% to 68% in the prevascular mediastinum. These are well-circumscribed heterogeneous masses, with variable contrast enhancement patterns. Punctate calcifications, and less commonly calcified phleboliths, may be identified.[51,52]

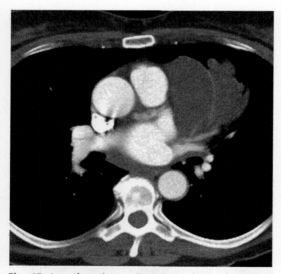

**Fig. 15.** Lymphangioma. Contrast-enhanced axial CT shows a left prevascular mediastinal multilocular cystic lesion with intrinsic septation. The lesion encases the left tracheobronchial tree and extends into the adjacent left upper lobe.

Dynamic contrast-enhanced (DCE) MR imaging may be utilized for further characterization.[53] Surgical excision can be both diagnostic and therapeutic.[52]

## THYMOLIPOMA

Thymolipomas are rare, benign, slow-growing thymic tumors that typically occur in young adults (mean age 27 years) but may affect patients over a wide age range, without gender predilection. Approximately 50% of patients are asymptomatic. When symptoms occur, they usually are secondary to compression of mediastinal structures.[54,55]

Thymolipomas usually are large, encapsulated, and composed of adipose and thymic tissue. On imaging, these tumors often manifest as large, prevascular mediastinal masses, most commonly in the inferior aspect of the mediastinum, and may be unilateral or bilateral. These tumors are soft and malleable, conform to the shape of adjacent structures, and may mimic cardiomegaly or diaphragmatic elevation on radiography. CT and MR imaging help establish a lesion's connection to the anatomic location of the thymus and demonstrate an admixture of fat and soft tissue components with a characteristic swirling morphology (**Fig. 16**). The fat component may be dominant, and such lesions may be indistinguishable from primary fat-containing neoplasms, such as lipomas. Complete surgical excision is curative.[54,55]

## LIPOMA AND LIPOSARCOMA

Lipomas are rare, benign, prevascular, mediastinal tumors comprising approximately 2% of all primary mediastinal neoplasms. On imaging, they typically manifest as well-circumscribed encapsulated lesions predominantly composed of fat, with a small amount of intrinsic soft tissue components and vascularity.[55]

Liposarcomas are even rarer and usually can be differentiated from lipomas due to a larger amount of intrinsic soft tissue and aggressive features, such as local invasion, mediastinal and/or hilar lymphadenopathy, or distant metastases (**Fig. 17**). Low-grade liposarcomas often are less heterogeneous in appearance and can be difficult to differentiate from lipomas.[56–58]

## MEDIASTINAL GOITER

Mediastinal goiter is one of the most frequently encountered mediastinal masses in clinical practice, with approximately 20% of thyroid goiters extending inferiorly into the mediastinum.[34] Although they typically affect asymptomatic

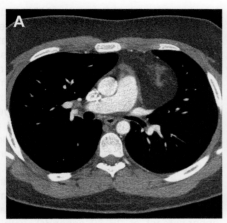
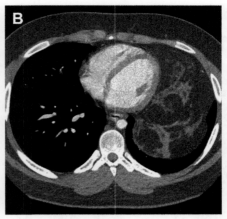

**Fig. 16.** Thymolipoma (*A, B*). Contrast-enhanced axial CT of the same patient at a more superior (*A*) and more inferior (*B*) level of the mediastinum shows a large heterogeneous mass in the left prevascular mediastinum that exhibits fat and soft tissue attenuation, corresponding to adipose and thymic tissue, respectively. Note the anatomic connection of the mass to the thymic bed (*A*), which strongly supports the diagnosis of thymolipoma.

women with palpable cervical goiters, they may produce symptoms of compression or pain.

Mediastinal goiters traditionally have been considered anterior mediastinal masses based on radiographic classification systems but may either descend into the prevascular mediastinal compartment or along the trachea into the visceral mediastinum. Primary intrathoracic or ectopic

thyroid goiters without a cervical component are rare.[34]

On radiography, mediastinal goiters frequently manifest with upper mediastinal widening and the characteristic cervicothoracic sign, which describes obscuration of the lesion's contours as it extends cephalad above the clavicle. This continuity between the cervical and mediastinal portions of the lesion is recognized easily on CT or MR imaging with multiplanar imaging. These usually are encapsulated, lobulated, and heterogenous masses with low attenuation foci that correspond to cyst formation and usually exhibit high attenuation due to iodine-containing portions of the gland. Calcifications are common and may be coarse, punctate, or ringlike. On contrast-enhanced CT, there is intense and sustained contrast enhancement[45] (**Fig. 18**). Nuclear scintigraphy with radioactive $^{123}$I and $^{131}$I can be diagnostic when functional thyroid tissue is present. Symptomatic patients and those with tumors of increasing heterogeneity or features suspicious for malignancy undergo surgical excision, with or without adjuvant or neoadjuvant $^{131}$I ablation in the setting of malignancy.

## MEDIASTINAL PARATHYROID ADENOMA

Parathyroid adenomas are benign functioning neoplasms that occur most commonly in the neck; however, approximately 10% are ectopic. Approximately 10% of all ectopic parathyroid adenomas occur in the prevascular mediastinum, usually near or within the thymus. These lesions most frequently affect older women, during the fifth to seventh decades of life, who often present with

**Fig. 17.** Liposarcoma. Contrast-enhanced coronal CT shows a large, predominantly fat attenuation mass involving the prevascular and visceral mediastinal compartments with intrinsic soft tissue components, exerting mass effect on surrounding structures, and extending into the neck. Tissue sampling confirmed liposarcoma.

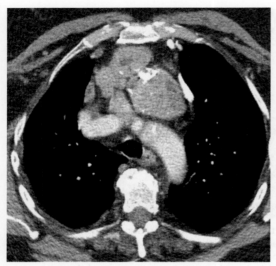

Fig. 18. Mediastinal goiter. Contrast-enhanced axial CT shows a large, lobulated, prevascular mediastinal goiter that demonstrates intense and sustained enhancement, cystic changes, and coarse calcifications. Multiplanar imaging (not shown) documented continuity with an enlarged cervical thyroid.

clinical hyperparathyroidism that persists after cervical parathyroidectomy.[59]

Parathyroid adenomas usually are small and encapsulated and measure less than 3 cm. On unenhanced CT, they are indistinguishable from

lymph nodes. Approximately 25% demonstrate contrast enhancement on contrast-enhanced CT[34] (Fig. 19). Ultrasound in combination with 99mTc sestamibi single-photon emission CT have been the modalities of choice for diagnosis and preoperative localization. Four-dimensional (4-D) CT acquiring images in 4 different phases (noncontrast, arterial, venous, and delayed), however, has shown higher sensitivity and accuracy for localization, characterization, and preoperative planning in ectopic adenomas. Multiplanar reformatted images and 3-dimensional volume-rendered images are reconstructed for optimal anatomic depiction. These lesions demonstrate intense enhancement in the arterial phase (peak enhancement at 25–60 seconds), with washout of contrast in the delayed phase; 4-D MR imaging, including unenhanced sequences and DCE, also is reliable for localization of parathyroid adenomas.[59,60]

## SUMMARY

Prevascular mediastinal masses include a wide range of benign and malignant entities. Although many mediastinal masses are discovered incidentally, affected patients may present with thoracic symptoms and/or with systemic effects of paraneoplastic syndromes or hormonal aberrations. Although the appearance of some prevascular mediastinal masses can be characteristic and diagnostic on CT, correlation with demographic information, clinical history, laboratory findings, and in some cases additional tests, such as MR imaging, FDG PET/CT, and nuclear scintigraphy, allows the formulation of a focused differential diagnosis and, in some cases, a specific diagnosis. Radiologists may use these methods to distinguish surgical from nonsurgical entities and thus inform appropriate patient management and impact outcomes. Treatment of choice varies based on the pathology, ranging from no intervention or serial imaging follow-up to surgical excision, chemotherapy, and/or radiation therapy.

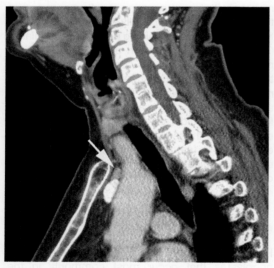

Fig. 19. Ectopic parathyroid adenoma. Contrast-enhanced 4-D sagittal CT (arterial phase) of a patient with primary hyperparathyroidism shows a small homogeneously enhancing soft tissue nodule (arrow) in the prevascular mediastinum which demonstrated uptake on Technetium-99m (99mTc) sestamibi scintigraphy (not shown), confirming parathyroid adenoma.

## CLINIC CARE POINTS

- When classic imaging features are present, a specific diagnosis may be suggested based solely on CT imaging features.
- Since appearance of various mediastinal lesions may overlap, additional imaging studies, laboratory tests, and tissue sampling often are required for a definitive diagnosis.
- Imaging cannot reliably definitively differentiate between thymomas, thymic carcinomas, and thymic neuroendocrine tumors.

## DISCLOSURE

The authors have nothing to disclose.

## REFERENCES

1. Felson B. Chest roentgenology. Philadelphia: WB Saunders; 1973.
2. Carter BW, Tomiyama N, Bhora FY, et al. A modern definition of mediastinal compartments. J Thorac Oncol 2014;9(9 Suppl 2):S97–101.
3. Takeda S-I, Miyoshi S, Akashi A, et al. Clinical spectrum of primary mediastinal tumors: a comparison of adult and pediatric populations at a single Japanese institution. J Surg Oncol 2003;83(1):24–30.
4. Carter BW, Benveniste MF, Marom EM, et al. Diagnostic approach to the anterior/prevascular mediastinum for radiologists. Mediastinum 2019;3:18.
5. Tomiyama N, Honda O, Tsubamoto M, et al. Anterior mediastinal tumors: diagnostic accuracy of CT and MRI. Eur J Radiol 2009;69(2):280–8.
6. Ackman JB, Wu CC. MRI of the thymus. AJR Am J Roentgenol 2011;197(1):W15–20.
7. Sung YM, Lee KS, Kim B-T, et al. 18F-FDG PET/CT of thymic epithelial tumors: usefulness for distinguishing and staging tumor subgroups. J Nucl Med 2006;47(10):1628–34.
8. Treglia G, Sadeghi R, Giovanella L, et al. Is (18)F-FDG PET useful in predicting the WHO grade of malignancy in thymic epithelial tumors? A meta-analysis. Lung Cancer 2014;86(1):5–13.
9. Luzzi L, Campione A, Gorla A, et al. Role of fluorine-flurodeoxyglucose positron emission tomography/computed tomography in preoperative assessment of anterior mediastinal masses. Eur J Cardiothorac Surg 2009;36(3):475–9.
10. Tatci E, Ozmen O, Dadali Y, et al. The role of FDG PET/CT in evaluation of mediastinal masses and neurogenic tumors of chest wall. Int J Clin Exp Med 2015;8(7):11146–52.
11. Jerushalmi J, Frenkel A, Bar-Shalom R, et al. Physiologic thymic uptake of 18F-FDG in children and young adults: a PET/CT evaluation of incidence, patterns, and relationship to treatment. J Nucl Med 2009;50(6):849–53.
12. Carter BW, Okumura M, Detterbeck FC, et al. Approaching the patient with an anterior mediastinal mass: a guide for radiologists. J Thorac Oncol 2014;9(9 Suppl 2):S110–8.
13. Inaoka T, Takahashi K, Mineta M, et al. Thymic hyperplasia and thymus gland tumors: differentiation with chemical shift MR imaging. Radiology 2007;243(3):869–76.
14. Carter BW, Benveniste MF, Madan R, et al. IASLC/ITMIG staging system and lymph node map for thymic epithelial neoplasms. Radiographics 2017;37(3):758–76.
15. Engels EA. Epidemiology of thymoma and associated malignancies. J Thorac Oncol 2010;5(10 Suppl 4):S260–5.
16. Johnson GB, Aubry MC, Yi ES, et al. Radiologic response to neoadjuvant treatment predicts histologic response in thymic epithelial tumors. J Thorac Oncol 2017;12(2):354–67.
17. Venuta F, Rendina EA, Anile M, et al. Thymoma and thymic carcinoma. Gen Thorac Cardiovasc Surg 2012;60(1):1–12.
18. Rosado-de-Christenson ML, Strollo DC. Marom EM Imaging of thymic epithelial neoplasms. Hematol Oncol Clin North Am 2008;22(3):409–31.
19. Duwe BV, Sterman DH. Musani AI Tumors of the mediastinum. Chest 2005;128(4):2893–909.
20. Strollo DC, Rosado-de-Christenson ML. Tumors of the thymus. J Thorac Imaging 1999;14(3):152–71.
21. Regnard JF, Magdeleinat P, Dromer C, et al. Prognostic factors and long-term results after thymoma resection: a series of 307 patients. J Thorac Cardiovasc Surg 1996;112(2):376–84.
22. Benveniste MFK, Rosado-de-Christenson ML, Sabloff BS, et al. Role of imaging in the diagnosis, staging, and treatment of thymoma. Radiographics 2011;31(7):1847–61 [discussion: 1861–3].
23. Shelly S, Agmon-Levin N, Altman A, et al. Thymoma and autoimmunity. Cell Mol Immunol 2011;8(3):199–202.
24. Bernard C, Frih H, Pasquet F, et al. Thymoma associated with autoimmune diseases: 85 cases and literature review. Autoimmun Rev 2016;15(1):82–92.
25. Tomiyama N, Müller NL, Ellis SJ, et al. Invasive and noninvasive thymoma: distinctive CT features. J Comput Assist Tomogr 2001;25(3):388–93.
26. Priola AM, Priola SM, Di Franco M, et al. Computed tomography and thymoma: distinctive findings in invasive and noninvasive thymoma and predictive features of recurrence. Radiol Med 2010;115(1):1–21.
27. Chaer R, Massad MG, Evans A, et al. Primary neuroendocrine tumors of the thymus. Ann Thorac Surg 2002;74(5):1733–40.
28. Gaur P, Leary C, Yao JC. Thymic neuroendocrine tumors: a SEER database analysis of 160 patients. Ann Surg 2010;251(6):1117–21.
29. Gibril F, Chen Y-J, Schrump DS, et al. Prospective study of thymic carcinoids in patients with multiple endocrine neoplasia type 1. J Clin Endocrinol Metab 2003;88(3):1066–81.
30. Fukai I, Masaoka A, Fujii Y, et al. Thymic neuroendocrine tumor (thymic carcinoid): a clinicopathologic study in 15 patients. Ann Thorac Surg 1999;67(1):208–11.
31. Piña-Oviedo S, Moran CA. Primary mediastinal classical hodgkin lymphoma. Adv Anat Pathol 2016;23(5):285–309.

32. Priola AM, Galetto G, Priola SM. Diagnostic and functional imaging of thymic and mediastinal involvement in lymphoproliferative disorders. Clin Imaging 2014;38(6):771–84.

33. Elstrom R, Guan L, Baker G, et al. Utility of FDG-PET scanning in lymphoma by WHO classification. Blood 2003;101(10):3875–6.

34. Strollo DC, Rosado-de-Christenson ML, Jett JR. Primary mediastinal tumors. Part 1: tumors of the anterior mediastinum. Chest 1997;112(2):511–22.

35. Moeller KH, Rosado-de-Christenson ML, Templeton PA. Mediastinal mature teratoma: imaging features. AJR Am J Roentgenol 1997;169(4):985–90.

36. Rodney AJ, Tannir NM, Siefker-Radtke AO, et al. Survival outcomes for men with mediastinal germ-cell tumors: the University of Texas M. D. Anderson Cancer Center experience. Urol Oncol 2012;30(6):879–85.

37. Dexeus FH, Logothetis CJ, Chong C, et al. Genetic abnormalities in men with germ cell tumors. J Urol 1988;140(1):80–4.

38. Nichols CR, Roth BJ, Heerema N, et al. Hematologic neoplasia associated with primary mediastinal germ-cell tumors. N Engl J Med 1990;322(20):1425–9.

39. Hartmann JT, Nichols CR, Droz JP, et al. Hematologic disorders associated with primary mediastinal nonseminomatous germ cell tumors. J Natl Cancer Inst 2000;92(1):54–61.

40. Bukowski RM, Wolf M, Kulander BG, et al. Alternating combination chemotherapy in patients with extragonadal germ cell tumors. A Southwest Oncology Group study. Cancer 1993;71(8):2631–8.

41. Nichols CR. Mediastinal germ cell tumors. Clinical features and biologic correlates. Chest 1991;99(2):472–9.

42. Lee KS, Im JG, Han CH, et al. Malignant primary germ cell tumors of the mediastinum: CT features. AJR Am J Roentgenol 1989;153(5):947–51.

43. Levitt RG, Husband JE, Glazer HS. CT of primary germ-cell tumors of the mediastinum. AJR Am J Roentgenol 1984;142(1):73–8.

44. Knapp RH, Hurt RD, Payne WS, et al. Malignant germ cell tumors of the mediastinum. J Thorac Cardiovasc Surg 1985;89(1):82–9.

45. Carter BW, Benveniste MF, Madan R, et al. ITMIG classification of mediastinal compartments and multidisciplinary approach to mediastinal masses. Radiographics 2017;37(2):413–36.

46. Takeda S-I, Miyoshi S, Minami M, et al. Clinical spectrum of mediastinal cysts. Chest 2003;124(1):125–32.

47. Wang X, Chen K, Li X, et al. Clinical features, diagnosis and thoracoscopic surgical treatment of thymic cysts. J Thorac Dis 2017;9(12):5203–11.

48. Choi YW, McAdams HP, Jeon SC, et al. Idiopathic multilocular thymic cyst: CT features with clinical and histopathologic correlation. AJR Am J Roentgenol 2001;177(4):881–5.

49. Bagrodia N, Defnet AM, Kandel JJ. Management of lymphatic malformations in children. Curr Opin Pediatr 2015;27(3):356–63.

50. Knight JK, Marshall. MB minimally invasive management of complex recurrent lymphangioma of the thorax and abdomen. Ann Thorac Surg 2016;101(6):e195–7.

51. Bai Y, Zhao G, Tan Y. CT and MRI manifestations of mediastinal cavernous hemangioma and a review of the literature. World J Surg Oncol 2019;17(1):205.

52. McAdams HP, Rosado-de-Christenson ML, Moran CA. Mediastinal hemangioma: radiographic and CT features in 14 patients. Radiology 1994;193(2):399–402.

53. Cheung YC, Ng SH, Wan YL, et al. Dynamic CT features of mediastinal hemangioma: more information for evaluation. J Clin Imaging 2000;24(5):276–8.

54. Rosado-de-Christenson ML, Pugatch RD, Moran CA, et al. Thymolipoma: analysis of 27 cases. Radiology 1994;193(1):121–6.

55. Gaerte SC, Meyer CA, Winer-Muram HT, et al. Fat-containing lesions of the chest. Radiographics 2002;22:S61–78. Spec No(suppl_1).

56. Munden RF, Nesbitt JC, Kemp BL, et al. Primary liposarcoma of the mediastinum. AJR Am J Roentgenol 2000;175(5):1340.

57. Munk PL, Lee MJ, Janzen DL, et al. Lipoma and liposarcoma: evaluation using CT and MR imaging. AJR Am J Roentgenol 1997;169(2):589–94.

58. Hahn HP. Fletcher CDM Primary mediastinal liposarcoma: clinicopathologic analysis of 24 cases. Am J Surg Pathol 2007;31(12):1868–74.

59. Argirò R, Diacinti D, Sacconi B, et al. Diagnostic accuracy of 3T magnetic resonance imaging in the preoperative localisation of parathyroid adenomas: comparison with ultrasound and 99mTc-sestamibi scans. Eur Radiol 2018;28(11):4900–8.

60. Ozturk M, Polat AV, Celenk C, et al. The diagnostic value of 4D MRI at 3T for the localization of parathyroid adenomas. Eur J Radiol 2019;112:207–13.

# Thymic Epithelial Neoplasms
## Radiologic-Pathologic Correlation

John P. Lichtenberger III, MD[a],*, Brett W. Carter, MD[b], Dane A. Fisher, MD[c], Regina F. Parker, MA/MBA[d], P. Gabriel Peterson, MD[e]

## KEYWORDS

- Thymic epithelial neoplasms • Thymoma • Radiologic-pathologic correlation
- Computed tomography • MR imaging

## KEY POINTS

- Thymic epithelial neoplasms, including thymoma, thymic carcinoma, and thymic carcinoid, are a rare group of tumors occurring in the anterior or prevascular mediastinum.
- Clinical presentations and syndromes associated with thymic epithelial neoplasms are important diagnostic clues to consider, and these clinical factors may ultimately guide management.
- The imaging features of these entities may overlap and an understanding of the radiologic-pathologic relationship helps clinical imagers arrive at the correct diagnosis and guide appropriate therapy.

## INTRODUCTION

Thymic epithelial neoplasms, as classified by the World Health Organization (WHO), include thymoma, thymic carcinoma, and thymic carcinoid. They are a rare group of tumors, and may be diagnosed incidentally, in the work-up of a parathymic syndrome, such as myasthenia gravis, or when mass effect or local invasion causes other symptoms. In each of these scenarios, understanding the radiologic-pathologic relationship of these neoplasms allows clinical imagers to contribute meaningfully to management decisions and overall patient care.

## THYMOMA
### Clinical Considerations

In adults older than the age of 40, thymomas are the most common neoplasm in prevascular mediastinum.[1] They are uncommon in children and adolescents. Thymomas account for approximately 80% of all thymic epithelial tumors and have no gender predilection.[2] Approximately one-third of patients are asymptomatic with many thymomas identified incidentally on thoracic imaging for other indications. However, depending on the size and location, thymomas can cause chest pain, dyspnea, cough, or phrenic nerve palsy. If the mass obstructs the superior vena cava, patients may develop symptoms, such as arm or facial swelling. The histologic components of thymomas also predispose patients to paraneoplastic syndromes, many of which are a result of autoimmune disorders and can result in a wide range of presenting symptomatology based on the associated abnormalities.

The thymus plays a key role in the developing immune system and is required for normal

[a] Department of Radiology, The George Washington University Medical Faculty Associates, 900 23rd Street, Northwest, Suite G 2092, Washington, DC 20037, USA; [b] Department of Thoracic Imaging, MD Anderson Cancer Center, 1515 Holcombe Boulevard, Unit 1478, Houston, TX 77030, USA; [c] Department of Radiology, Naval Medical Center Portsmouth, 620 John Paul Jones Circle, Portsmouth, VA 23708, USA; [d] Harvard Medical School, 25 Shattuck Street, Boston, MA 02115, USA; [e] Department of Radiology, Walter Reed National Military Medical Center, 8901 Rockville Pike, Bethesda, MD 20889, USA
* Corresponding author. 1914 Stratton Road, Silver Spring, MD 20910.
E-mail address: jlichtenberger@mfa.gwu.edu

Radiol Clin N Am 59 (2021) 169–182
https://doi.org/10.1016/j.rcl.2020.11.005
0033-8389/21/© 2020 Elsevier Inc. All rights reserved.

maturation of T lymphocytes. This maturation process relies on normal thymic architecture. Although most thymomas occur in adults after the normal thymus has involuted, they can produce and release immature T lymphocytes into systemic circulation. Without the normal architecture of the thymus to filter out abnormal or self-reactive T lymphocytes, these immature cells may result in autoimmune disorders. The amount and type of lymphocytes produced varies by subtype of thymoma.[3]

The most frequent paraneoplastic autoimmune syndrome associated with thymoma is myasthenia gravis (Table 1). One-third to one-half of patients with thymoma have myasthenia gravis[3–5] and in most cases there are abnormal antibodies directed toward acetylcholine receptors.[6] Conversely, only 10% to 20% of patients with myasthenia gravis have a thymoma.[7–9] Regardless, patients who present with myasthenia gravis should be screened for thymoma at diagnosis.[7] Other, less common paraneoplastic syndromes associated with thymoma include hypogamma-globulinemia in 5% to 20%, pure red cell aplasia in approximately 4%, and neuromyotonia (Isaac syndrome) in 3%.[10]

Numerous categorization systems have been developed for thymoma, which has resulted in significant interobserver variability regarding how these tumors have been classified, staged, and treated over time. The Masaoka clinical staging system, first proposed in 1981, is an excellent predictor of prognosis for thymoma but is not as well suited for thymic carcinomas.[2,11] Subsequently, a preliminary tumor-node-metastasis (TNM) classification system was proposed in 1991 and a modified classification by Koga and colleagues in 1994.[12,13] The Masaoka-Koga modified classification system is characterized by the following features[13,14]:

- Stage I: Grossly and microscopically completely encapsulated tumor
- Stage IIa: Microscopic transcapsular invasion
- Stage IIb: Macroscopic invasion into thymic or surrounding fatty tissue, or grossly adherent to but not breaking through mediastinal pleura or pericardium
- Stage III: Macroscopic invasion into neighboring organ, such as the great vessels, pericardium, or lung
- Stage IVa: Pleural or pericardial dissemination
- Stage IVb: Lymphogenous or hematogenous metastasis

In the most recent 2017 American Joint Committee on Cancer TNM (eighth edition) system for thymomas, staging is based on local invasion, lymph node involvement, and metastasis.[15] The T categories are determined by the presence or absence of invasion and, if present, what surrounding structures are involved.[16] The incidence of lymph node involvement or distant metastasis in thymoma is less than 5%.[2] When lymph node involvement does occur from thymoma, it is localized to the prevascular mediastinum 90% of the time. The currently accepted method for describing lymph node involvement from thymoma is separated into two groups, anterior and deep, according to the proposed lymph node mapping schema developed by the ITMIG/IASLC project.[17] When distant metastasis is present, it is grouped into pleural/pericardial or distant.[18]

## Pathologic Features

The most widely used histologic classification system is the WHO fourth edition published in 2015 by Travis and colleagues,[19] which is summarized next. There are five main subtypes of thymomas: type A, AB, B1, B2, and B3. Other recognized subtypes of thymomas include micronodular thymoma with lymphoid stroma, metaplastic thymoma, microscopic thymoma, sclerosing thymoma, and lipofibroadenoma. Because thymomas are frequently composed of several subtypes, it is now recommended to include all identified subtypes in the pathologic report (except for type AB thymomas, which are already a combination of types A and B by definition) in order of predominance by 10% increments.[20] The 2015 WHO classification system also includes immunohistochemistry, which may help differentiate thymomas with otherwise ambiguous histology (Figs. 1–3).

Type A thymomas are also known as spindle cell thymomas and are uncommon, accounting for less than 15% of all thymomas. They are generally well circumscribed or encapsulated and composed of spindle or oval tumor cells with few if any immature lymphocytes. Common histopathologic growth patterns include rosettes, glandular or glomeruloid appearance with occasional microcystic change peripherally. Mitotic activity tends to be low. Atypical type A thymoma variant is a recognized entity with some degree of atypia or increased mitotic activity.

Type AB thymomas are more common, accounting for approximately 25% of all thymomas and are distinguished by their morphology and the number of immature lymphocytes. AB thymomas have a lymphocyte-poor spindle cell component (type A) and a lymphocyte-rich component (type B) and a significant number of immature

**Table 1**
Thymic epithelial neoplasms[a]

| Subtypes | 5-y Survival | Histopathology | Imaging | Associated Syndromes |
|---|---|---|---|---|
| *Thymomas[b] (>70%) adults 50–60 y with wide range* | | | | |
| Type A | 100% | Spindloid epithelial cells with rare to no lymphocytes | CT (commonly): Homogenously enhancing, unilateral lobulated mass with smooth margins and fibrous capsule; completely or partially outlined by fat | Myasthenia gravis (35%); hypogammaglobulinemia (5%–20%); red cell aplasia (4%); neuromyotonia (3%) |
| Type AB | 100% | Spindloid epithelial cells admixed with lymphocyte-rich foci, either diffusely or in discrete nodules | CT (rarely): Heterogeneously enhancing mass arising anywhere from lower neck to cardiophrenic borders with loculations; cystic components; curvilinear or punctate calcifications; irregular margins; local invasion; mediastinal adenopathy; and metastases (<5%) to pleura/pericardium | |
| Type B1 | 95% | Polygonal epithelial cells forming anastomosing network obscured by normal thymic architecture with diffuse lymphocytes | | |
| Type B2 | 95% | Polygonal epithelial cells in clusters with diffuse lymphocyte-rich background; possible palisading of tumor cells along perivascular spaces; epithelial cell nuclei large and vesicular with prominent nucleoli | MR imaging: Intermediate T1 and hyperintense T2, with hypointense internal fibrous septa and fibrous capsule; CSR[c] >1.0 | |
| Type B3 | 92% | Polygonal epithelial cells with mild-to-moderate atypia forming confluent sheets with rare lymphocytes; epithelial cell nuclei moderate in size | FDG PET/CT: Low or variable FDG uptake; $SUV_{max}{}^d$ <11.6 SSTR (+) | |
| *Thymic carcinoma (20%) adults older than 50 y* | | | | |
| Type C | 38% | Clear-cut cytologic atypia with cytoarchitecture dissimilar to normal thymus; range of morphologic subtypes[f] | CT: Heterogeneously enhancing mass with loculations; calcifications (10%–61%); irregular margins; local invasion; and distant metastases (50%–65%) to brain, bone, lung, and liver MR imaging: Solid components hyperintense on T1 and T2; CSR >1.0; ADC[e] values <1.56 × $10^{-3}$ $mm^2$/s FDG PET/CT: High FDG uptake $SUV_{max}$ >11.6 SSTR (+) | Rarely: Myasthenia gravis; red cell aplasia; hypogammaglobulinemia |

(continued on next page)

**Table 1**
*(continued)*

| Subtypes | 5-y Survival | Histopathology | Imaging | Associated Syndromes |
|---|---|---|---|---|
| *Thymic carcinoid tumor (2%–5%)* *Male (3:1) adults 40–60 y with wide range* | | | | |
| Typical | 50%–100% | Predominantly or exclusively neuroendocrine cells marked by diffuse expression of neuroendocrine markers[g] in 50% of tumor cells; low (typical) or intermediate (atypical) grade; range of histologic subtypes[h] | CT: Heterogeneously enhancing unencapsulated mass with possible calcifications; irregular margins; local invasion; and distant metastases (20%–40%) to skin, adrenal glands, bone, lung, pleura, brain, or kidney. MR imaging: Heterogenous hyperintensity on T2 FDG PET/CT: High FDG uptake SSTR (++) MIBG (+) | Functional activity (33%–50%) resulting in endocrinopathies (Cushing syndrome in 40%; SIADH; carcinoid syndrome in 2%) Rarely: MEN type 1 (25%) and 2 |
| Atypical | 20%–80% | | | |

*Abbreviations:* CSR, chemical shift ratio; CT, computed tomography; FDG, fluorodeoxyglucose; MEN, multiple neuroendocrine neoplasia; MIBG, I-131 or I-123 metaiodobenzylguanidine imaging; SIADH, syndrome of inappropriate antidiuretic hormone secretion; SSTR, somatostatin receptor imaging with In-111 pentetreotide or Ga-68 DOTATATE; SUV, standardized uptake value.

  a  Excluding rare neoplasms, including high-grade thymic neuroendocrine tumors (small cell carcinoma; large cell neuroendocrine carcinoma) and thymic teratoma.

  b  (A) Excluding rare types of thymomas, including micronodular thymoma with lymphoid stroma, metaplastic thymoma, microscopic thymoma, sclerosing thymoma, lipofibroadenoma, and atypical type A variant. (B) More than 50% of thymomas are classified as multiple subtypes. Estimated prevalence of each subtype: type A (4%–7%), type AB (28%–34%), type B1 (9%–20%), type B2 (20%–36%), and type B3 (10%–14%).

  c  Chemical shift MR imaging may distinguish benign (CSR <0.7) from neoplastic (CSR >1.0) tissue. CSR is derived from dual-echo, single breath-hold gradient echo T1-weighted imaging with in-phase (IP) and opposed-phase (OP) images. CSR = [(thymus OP/muscle OP)/(thymus IP/muscle IP)].

  d  ¹⁸FDG PET/CT maximum SUV may distinguish thymoma (SUV$_{max}$ <11.6) from thymic carcinoma (SUV$_{max}$ >11.6).

  e  ADC values >1.56 × 10⁻³ mm²/s predict that a tumor is benign with 94% specificity, and higher ADC values correspond to well-differentiated tumors.

  f  Subtypes include squamous (most common), mucoepidermoid, lymphoepithelioma-like, clear cell, basaloid, adenocarcinoma, papillary, rhabdoid, hepatoid, rhabdomyomatous, sarcomatoid, and undifferentiated/anaplastic.

  g  Neuroendocrine markers include synaptophysin, chromogranin, CD56, and neuron-specific enolase.

  h  Subtypes include classic carcinoid, spindle cell, pigmented, oncocytic/oxyphilic, mucinous, angiomatoid, carcinoid with sarcomatous change, and carcinoid with amyloid.

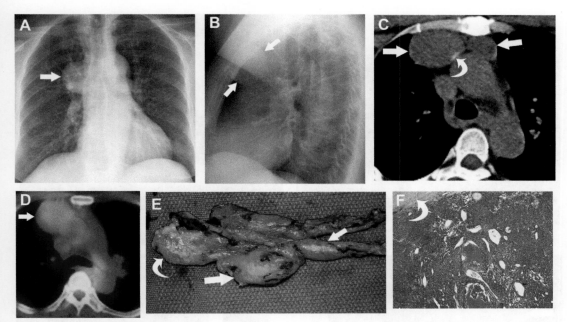

**Fig. 1.** A 64-year-old woman with WHO type A thymoma. (*A*) Frontal chest radiograph shows a well-defined opacity (*arrow*) projecting over the right hilum (the so-called "hilum overlay" sign), suggesting localization to the anterior mediastinum. (*B*) Lateral chest radiograph confirms anterior mediastinal location of the mass (*arrows*) with well-defined superior and inferior borders. (*C*) Unenhanced axial CT shows a bilobed soft tissue mass (*straight arrows*) with peripheral calcification (*curved arrow*) in the prevascular mediastinum. (*D*) Fused axial fluorodeoxyglucose PET/computed tomography shows increased fluorodeoxyglucose uptake in the mass (*arrow*). (*E*) Gross specimen shows an encapsulated, bilobed mass (*straight arrows*) with adjacent mediastinal fat (*curved arrow*). (*F*) Photomicrograph (hematoxylin-eosin, original magnification ×40) shows a proliferation of spindle-shaped, elongated cells, bland nuclei without atypia. The capsule (*curved arrow*) is preserved.

lymphocytes. The overall tumor is also typically encapsulated with multiple lobulations. The discrete A and B components may form separate nodules or be intermixed throughout the mass.

Type B1 thymomas account for approximately 20% of all thymomas. They resemble normal thymus architecture including medullary differentiation and an immature lymphocyte-rich background. Type B2 thymomas account for an average of 25% of all thymomas. Histopathologically they are lymphocyte-rich with a lobular organization and fibrous capsule and interspersed polygonal neoplastic thymic epithelial cells, which are usually in clusters. Type B3 thymomas account for approximately 15% of all thymomas. In type B3 thymomas there is a predominance of moderately atypical polygonal epithelial cells forming solid sheets and few immature lymphocytes.

Given the wide range of clinical behavior that is possible for all subtypes of thymoma, clinical staging carries much more prognostic significance.[21] Involvement of the surrounding fatty mediastinal tissue carries the same prognosis as an encapsulated tumor as long as there is no invasion of the mediastinal pleura.[22] It is also worth noting that pathologic specimens must be handled carefully to preserve

the loose surrounding connective tissue, which is critical to pathologic staging.[22] If the patient received preoperative neoadjuvant chemotherapy, there are variable treatment-related changes that seem to depend on the tumor subtype and should be described in the pathology report.[23]

## Imaging Features

The thymus is a bilobed triangular structure located in the prevascular mediastinum.[24–26] Before assessing thymoma, normal residual thymus or benign thymic hyperplasia must be excluded. There is a general trend of fatty replacement of the thymus with age, generally beginning after puberty, but with a wide degree of variability. In a retrospective cohort study of more than 2500 patients, approximately 75% of patients with a mean age of 58 had complete fatty replacement of the thymus.[27] There are also differences between male and female thymic attenuation with increased thymic attenuation in females relative to males in the 20 to 30 year age range.[28]

Computed tomography (CT) of the chest is the imaging modality of choice for the evaluation of thymoma with the primary goals being detection

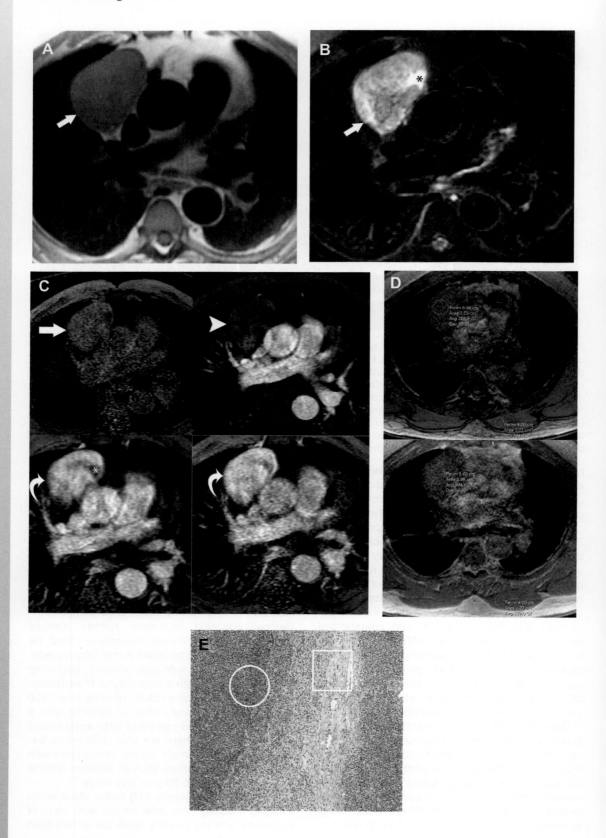

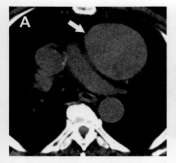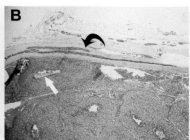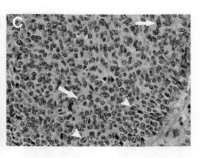

Fig. 3. A 74-year-old man with WHO type B3 thymoma. (A) Unenhanced axial CT demonstrates a well-circumscribed mass (arrow) in the left prevascular mediastinum with attenuation slightly higher than skeletal muscle. Fat planes are preserved around the encapsulated mass. (B) Photomicrograph (hematoxylin-eosin, original magnification ×40) shows multiple areas of necrosis (straight arrow) and capsular invasion (curved arrow). (C) Photomicrograph (hematoxylin-eosin, original magnification ×40) demonstrates cellular atypia (straight arrows), multiple mitoses (arrowheads), and few lymphocytes.

of local invasion and identification of distant metastasis.[29] Invasion is a critical component of the T staging category, but it is difficult to reliably identify on imaging (**Figs. 4** and **5**).[30] For this reason, intravenous contrast should be administered to optimize evaluation for vascular invasion, which characterizes T3/T4 disease. Local or distant nodal involvement with short-axis dimension greater than 1 cm should be identified and reported in the context of the ITMIG/IASLC lymph node mapping project for thymic epithelial neoplasms.[17]

On CT, thymomas typically arise from one lobe of the thymus and therefore tend to be unilateral lobulated masses in the prevascular compartment.[29] Thymomas less commonly occur in the cardiophrenic angles or along the cardiac borders.[24] Although thymomas are most commonly homogeneously solid in attenuation, they may have cystic components or calcifications, which are usually linear and peripheral but can also be distributed throughout the mass.[31] If present, surrounding infiltration of mediastinal fat should be described; however, encapsulated tumors and those with extension limited to mediastinal fat are characterized as T1 lesions. Irregular margins or frank invasion into the pericardium, lung, vasculature, chest wall, myocardium, trachea, or esophagus must be described because all carry implications for T status. If there is possible vascular invasion, the specific vessels involved should be detailed because involvement of the brachiocephalic vein, superior vena cava, or extrapericardial pulmonary vasculature is classified as T3, whereas involvement of the aorta, arch vessels, or intrapericardial pulmonary artery is classified as T4. Diaphragmatic elevation is a pertinent associated finding because this could suggest phrenic nerve involvement (T3).

Lymph nodes greater than 1 cm short-axis in either the anterior or deep compartments should be described in the context of the ITMIG/IASLC lymph node mapping project.[17] Extensive mediastinal lymphadenopathy should raise suspicion for alternate diagnoses, such as thymic carcinoma, lymphoma, lung cancer, or metastatic disease.[29] Although discrete pleural or pericardial nodules separate from the primary tumor suggest drop

Fig. 2. A 65-year-old man with WHO type AB thymoma. (A) Axial T1 double inversion recovery (DIR) MR image shows a well-circumscribed mass in the prevascular mediastinum (arrow) with preservation of adjacent fat planes. (B) Axial T2 DIR MR image with fat saturation shows a heterogeneously hyperintense mass (arrow) without evidence of adjacent organ invasion. Some regions of high signal intensity are consistent with fluid components (asterisk). (C) Composite axial three-dimensional spoiled gradient echo pulse sequence images with fat suppression without and with intravenous gadolinium contrast shows that the prevascular mass on the precontrast image (straight arrow) demonstrates no arterial enhancement (arrowhead) and progressive heterogeneous enhancement on delayed sequences (curved arrows). The nonenhancing regions (asterisk) indicate fluid or necrosis. (D) Axial dual-echo, single breath-hold gradient echo T1-weighted chemical shift MR images with in-phase (bottom) and out-of-phase (top) show a chemical shift ratio of 0.8. (E) Photomicrograph (hematoxylin-eosin, original magnification ×40) shows a lymphocyte-rich component (circle) and a spindle cell–predominant component (square) of a WHO type AB thymoma.

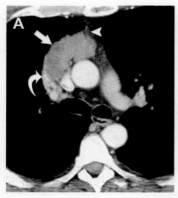
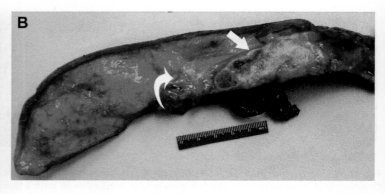
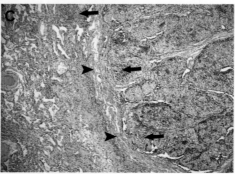

**Fig. 4.** A 53-year-old man with invasive thymoma. (*A*) Contrast-enhanced axial CT shows a heterogeneous prevascular mass (*straight arrow*) with compression of the adjacent lung (*curved arrow*) and loss of the fat plane between the mass and the lung, indicating invasion (*arrowhead*). A subtle focus of high attenuation is present in the adjacent mediastinal fat, suggesting mediastinal fat invasion confirmed at surgery. (*B*) Gross specimen shows the mass (*straight arrow*) invading the adjacent lung (*curved arrow*). (*C*) Photomicrograph (hematoxylin-eosin, original magnification ×40) shows tumor cells (*arrows*) invading the lung parenchyma (*arrowheads*).

metastases (M1a disease), pulmonary parenchymal nodules are more common in thymic carcinoma or lung cancer rather than thymoma.

MR imaging is useful in evaluating indeterminate prevascular mediastinal masses and can often distinguish between benign residual thymus or thymic hyperplasia and thymic neoplasm. A chemical shift ratio of 0.7 or less and a signal intensity index greater than 8.9% on MR imaging are consistent with benign thymic tissue or thymic hyperplasia.[32,33] These values are derived from signal intensities measured on dual-echo, single breath-hold gradient echo T1-weighted chemical shift MR imaging with in-phase (IP) and opposed-phase (OP) images. The chemical shift ratio is defined as [(Thymus OP/Muscle OP)/(Thymus IP/Muscle IP)] and the signal intensity index is defined as [(Thymus IP – Thymus OP)/(Thymus IP) * 100%.

On MR imaging, thymomas are most commonly low-to-intermediate signal intensity on T1-weighted imaging and hyperintense on T2-weighted imaging, occasionally with visualization of hypointense internal fibrous septa and a fibrous capsule.[34,35] There is increasing evidence that diffusion-weighted imaging and dynamic contrast-enhanced MR imaging may aid in the differentiation of benign versus malignant mediastinal lesions.[36]

Fluorodeoxyglucose (FDG) PET/CT has a limited role in the evaluation of thymoma. Thymomas can have variable metabolic activity denoted by standardized uptake value (SUV) but higher SUV values are suggestive of thymic carcinoma or thymic carcinoid. Overall, there have been mixed results in studies attempting to differentiate low-risk from high-risk thymomas, B2 and B3 according to the Masaoka-Koga classification system.[37,38]

## Management

All subtypes of thymoma can behave aggressively and should no longer be called benign according to the most recent WHO classification.[20] The ITMIG recommends extended thymectomy including resection of prevascular mediastinal lymph nodes for all thymomas and sampling of deep lymph nodes when

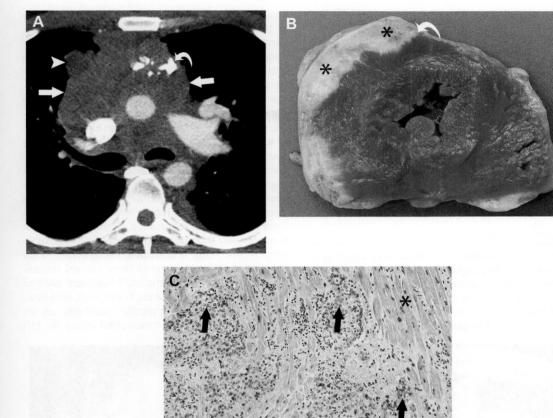

**Fig. 5.** A 38-year-old man with invasive thymoma. (*A*) Contrast-enhanced axial CT demonstrates a large, heterogeneous mediastinal mass (*straight arrows*) centered in the prevascular mediastinum and invading multiple mediastinal structures, evidenced by obliteration of fat planes adjacent to the aorta and pulmonary arteries. Internal calcification (*curved arrow*) and cystic spaces (*arrowhead*) are present. (*B*) Sectioned gross specimen shows the mass (*asterisks*) invading the myocardium (*curved arrow*) of the left ventricle. (*C*) Photomicrograph (hematoxylin-eosin, original magnification ×40) demonstrates tumor cells (*arrows*) invading the myocardium (*asterisks*).

thymomas invade adjacent structures.[39] Because achieving complete surgical resection improves survival regardless of stage or histologic classification, neoadjuvant chemotherapy may be used to convert unresectable tumors into resectable tumors.[40] When there are positive margins or evidence of microscopic invasion into surrounding tissue on the pathologic specimen, adjuvant radiation therapy is indicated. Thymectomy is also recommended for patients with nonthymomatous myasthenia gravis with improved outcomes possibly related to the immunologic role of the thymus discussed previously.[9]

## THYMIC CARCINOMA
### Clinical Considerations

Thymic carcinoma is a malignant neoplasm that arises from thymic epithelial cells and accounts for 20% of thymic epithelial neoplasms.[41] The average age of diagnosis is 50 years with men and women equally affected.[41] Patients most commonly present with symptoms of mediastinal mass effect, superior vena cava syndrome, or invasion of mediastinal structures.[42] Although paraneoplastic syndromes are rare, myasthenia gravis, pure red cell aplasia, and hypogammaglobulinemia can occur in thymic carcinoma.[42]

## Pathologic Features

Thymic carcinoma arises from thymic epithelial cells. The current WHO classification system is based on histologic findings with thymic carcinoma representing a type C tumor.[24] Neoplastic epithelial cells show overt morphologic and immunohistochemical atypia, which are features seen in carcinomas of other organs (**Fig. 6**).[41,43] Other histologic features include an infiltrative growth pattern, tumor cell nests in desmoplastic stroma, and lack of immature T cells.[43] Squamous cell carcinoma is the most common subtype of thymic carcinoma with several other less common subtypes described.[20,42]

## Imaging Features

Thymoma and thymic carcinoma have significant overlap in imaging features and are therefore often indistinguishable based on imaging alone.[44] Thymic carcinoma is often initially detected on chest radiography as a nonspecific anterior mediastinal mass. CT typically shows a prevascular soft

tissue attenuation mass of variable size. Because of the embryologic development of the thymus, carcinoma can also be found in a variety of locations to include the junction of the great vessels and pericardium, cardiophrenic angles, heart borders, neck, and other mediastinal compartments.[24] Tumor attenuation is variable depending on associated hemorrhage and necrosis. Calcifications can also be seen in 10% to 61% of tumors on CT.[45] Although there is considerable overlap with thymoma, lobulations, irregular borders, and invasion of adjacent fat and vessels are more aggressive features that suggest a diagnosis of thymic carcinoma.[24,36] These findings also correlate with a higher likelihood of metastasis and disease recurrence. Thymic carcinoma is more likely than thymoma to cause mediastinal lymphadenopathy and distant metastasis.[36] Fifty percent to 65% of patients have distant metastasis at the time of diagnosis.[41] Frequent sites of metastasis include the brain, bone, lung, and liver.

Thymic carcinoma typically manifests as an enhancing prevascular mediastinal mass on MR

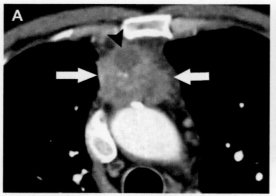
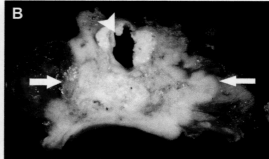
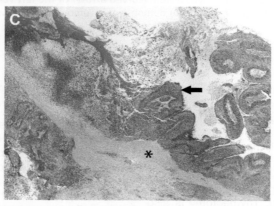

**Fig. 6.** A 61-year-old man with thymic carcinoma. (*A*) Contrast-enhanced axial CT demonstrates a heterogeneous prevascular mass (*arrows*) with mediastinal fat invasion and an internal fluid component (*arrowhead*) consistent with a cyst or necrosis. (*B*) Sectioned gross specimen shows the tumor infiltrating the mediastinal fat (*arrows*) with central necrosis (*arrowhead*). (*C*) Photomicrograph (hematoxylin-eosin, original magnification ×40) shows carcinomatous (*arrow*) and sarcomatoid (*asterisk*) components and areas of necrosis. Necrosis is more common in thymic carcinoma than thymoma.

imaging. Solid components of the tumor are typically hyperintense on T1-weighted and T2-weighted images.[41] More aggressive features, such as lobulations, invasion of adjacent structures, and lesion heterogeneity, may be seen. Hemorrhage, necrosis, flow voids, and calcifications can all cause low T2 signal within the mass. These heterogeneous features in conjunction with mediastinal lymphadenopathy may favor a diagnosis of thymic carcinoma.[46] Low ADC values suggest increased tumor aggressiveness and poor differentiation.[36]

FDG PET/CT is useful for differentiating thymic carcinoma from thymoma and other thymic masses and pseudomasses.[24] Thymic carcinoma typically has a higher degree of FDG-avid disease compared with thymoma with good sensitivity and specificity when using SUVmax greater than 5.[47,48] FDG PET/CT may also be performed to evaluate for metastatic disease and monitor response to therapy.

## Management

Thymic carcinoma has a worse prognosis and higher recurrence rate than thymoma. The 5-year survival rate for thymic carcinoma is 30% to 50% and recurrence rate is high even following complete resection.[42] Standard management of thymic carcinoma is based on the resectability of the tumor at initial diagnosis. For resectable tumors, surgical excision is first performed followed by chemotherapy and radiation.[49] Neoadjuvant chemotherapy with or without radiotherapy is used for tumors determined to be initially nonresectable.[49] Following this therapy, the tumor is surgically removed with additional postsurgical radiotherapy. Postoperative chemotherapy may also be used. Palliative chemotherapy is reserved for patients with metastatic disease. Immunotherapy is an emerging treatment of thymic carcinoma refractory to the standard therapies described previously.[49] Because PD-1 and/or PD-L1 are expressed in most thymic epithelial neoplasms, this marker serves as a target for PD-1 inhibitors, such as pembrolizumab and nivolumab; however, patients must be monitored closely for the development of severe autoimmune disorders.[49]

## THYMIC CARCINOID TUMOR
### Clinical Considerations

Thymic carcinoid tumor is a subtype of thymic neuroendocrine tumor. It is a rare and predominantly low-grade malignancy that accounts for 2% to 5% of thymic epithelial neoplasms.[50] This tumor is found more commonly in men at a 3:1 ratio and has a wide age range with median age of 43 years.[24,41] One-third of thymic carcinoid tumors are functional,

causing endocrine disorders, such as Cushing syndrome and multiple endocrine neoplasia.[41] Most patients present with symptoms from mass effect or mediastinal invasion.

### Pathologic Features

Thymic carcinoid tumors are unencapsulated tumors predominantly or exclusively composed of neuroendocrine cells.[50] Thymic carcinoid tumors do not show organ-specific histology or immunohistochemistry, which makes relevant clinical and radiologic information essential for accurate diagnosis.[51] The 2015 WHO classification system categorizes typical and atypical carcinoid tumors as subtypes of thymic neuroendocrine tumors, which are considered low- and intermediate-grade tumors, respectively.[20] These subtypes are differentiated histologically by the number of mitoses and absence or presence of necrosis. Large cell neuroendocrine carcinoma and small cell carcinoma represent the high-grade subtypes of thymic neuroendocrine tumor.[20] Immunohistochemical staining can show expression of synaptophysin, chromogranin, CD56, and neuron-specific enolase. Neuroendocrine differentiation is defined by diffuse expression of at least one of these markers in greater than 50% of tumor cells.[20]

### Imaging Features

Thymic carcinoid tumor has a nonspecific appearance on imaging that can overlap with thymoma and thymic carcinoma. Chest radiography may show an anterior mediastinal mass or be normal. On cross-sectional imaging, typical features include a large, heterogeneously enhancing prevascular mass with irregular borders and local invasion.[50] MR imaging shows heterogeneous T2 hyperintense signal.[50] There is no fibrous capsule.[41] Atypical carcinoid tumor is prone to hemorrhage and necrosis. These tumors show aggressive features, such as invasion of adjacent mediastinal structures and metastasis to mediastinal lymph nodes and distant sites.[52] One small study showed internal calcifications in 9% of tumors.[50] Occasionally, a thymic mass may be occult even in the setting of endocrine abnormalities.[41] Thymic carcinoid tumor and metastatic disease are typically FDG avid on PET/CT. Thymic carcinoid shows similar radiotracer uptake on I-123 and I-131 MIBG as carcinoid tumors of other organ systems.[53] Somatostatin receptor imaging is also sensitive for the identification of thymic carcinoid tumor.[54] For all neuroendocrine tumors, Ga-68 DOTATATE PET/CT provides a high diagnostic sensitivity of 87.1% to 90.9%.[55] In-111 Octreoscan demonstrates a lower sensitivity of

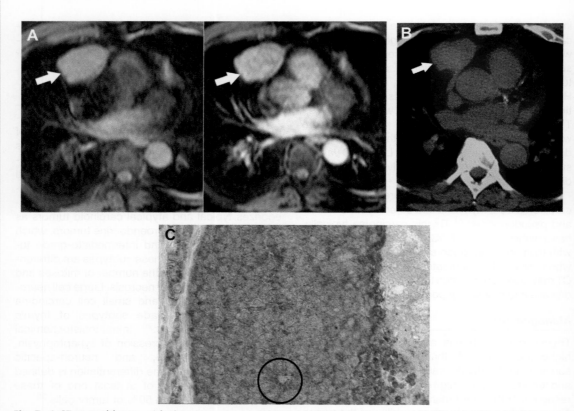

**Fig. 7.** A 67-year-old man with thymic carcinoid. (*A*) Axial T1 MR images without (*left*) and with (*right*) intravenous gadolinium contrast demonstrate an intrinsically hyperintense mass (*arrow*) relative to skeletal muscle with faint internal enhancement. (*B*) Axial In-111 octreoscan single-photon emission CT/CT shows focal radiotracer uptake in the mass (*arrow*), consistent with somatostatin receptor expression seen in neuroendocrine tumors. (*C*) Photomicrograph (synaptophysin, original magnification ×40) shows diffuse staining of tumor cells and a rosette pattern (*circle*), consistent with neuroendocrine origin.

35% to 80%.[56] The sensitivity of somatostatin receptor imaging is dependent on tumor type, size, and expression of somatostatin receptors (**Fig. 7**).[55]

## Management

The reported 5-year survival rates for typical and atypical carcinoid are 50% to 100% and 20% to 80%, respectively.[51] Higher grade tumors have a poor prognosis because of a high rate of recurrence and metastasis. The primary method of management is aggressive surgical resection of the primary tumor, which at times involves resection of the pleura, pericardium, and great vessels.[57] Local disease without nodal or distant metastasis is typically treated with surgery alone.[54] The National Cancer Comprehensive Network guidelines recommend chemotherapy with or without radiation in patients with unresectable or metastatic disease; however, there is variability in the reported effectiveness of these additional treatment strategies.[57]

## SUMMARY

Thymic epithelial neoplasms are an important consideration when prevascular mediastinal masses are identified on imaging examinations. Integrating important imaging features, such as local invasion, and pathologic features, such as necrosis and immunohistochemistry, ensures a meaningful contribution by clinical imagers to the care team.

## DISCLOSURE

J.P. Lichtenberger: Elsevier. D.A. Fisher, R.F. Parker, P.G. Peterson: The opinions and assertions contained herein are the private views of the authors and are not to be construed as official nor as representing the views of the Departments of the Army, Navy, Air Force, or Defense.

## REFERENCES

1. Strollo DC, Rosado de Christenson ML, Jett JR. Primary mediastinal tumors. Part 1: tumors of the anterior mediastinum. Chest 1997;112(2):511–22.

2. Kondo K. Tumor-node metastasis staging system for thymic epithelial tumors. J Thorac Oncol 2010;5(10 Suppl 4):S352–6.

3. Weksler B, Lu B. Alterations of the immune system in thymic malignancies. J Thorac Oncol 2014;9(9 Suppl 2):S137–42.

4. Lewis JE, Wick MR, Scheithauer BW, et al. Thymoma. A clinicopathologic review. Cancer 1987; 60(11):2727–43.

5. Mygland A, Vincent A, Newsom-Davis J, et al. Autoantibodies in thymoma-associated myasthenia gravis with myositis or neuromyotonia. Arch Neurol 2000;57(4):527–31.

6. Meriggioli MN, Sanders DB. Muscle autoantibodies in myasthenia gravis: beyond diagnosis? Expert Rev Clin Immunol 2012;8(5):427–38.

7. Evoli A, Lancaster E. Paraneoplastic disorders in thymoma patients. J Thorac Oncol 2014;9(9 Suppl 2):S143–7.

8. Marx A, Pfister F, Schalke B, et al. The different roles of the thymus in the pathogenesis of the various myasthenia gravis subtypes. Autoimmun Rev 2013; 12(9):875–84.

9. Wolfe GI, Kaminski HJ, Aban IB, et al. Randomized trial of thymectomy in myasthenia gravis. N Engl J Med 2016;375(6):511–22.

10. Marx A, Willcox N, Leite MI, et al. Thymoma and paraneoplastic myasthenia gravis. Autoimmunity 2010; 43(5–6):413–27.

11. Masaoka A, Monden Y, Nakahara K, et al. Follow-up study of thymomas with special reference to their clinical stages. Cancer 1981;48(11):2485–92.

12. Yamakawa Y, Masaoka A, Hashimoto T, et al. A tentative tumor-node-metastasis classification of thymoma. Cancer 1991;68(9):1984–7.

13. Koga K, Matsuno Y, Noguchi M, et al. A review of 79 thymomas: modification of staging system and reappraisal of conventional division into invasive and non-invasive thymoma. Pathol Int 1994;44(5): 359–67.

14. Detterbeck FC, Nicholson AG, Kondo K, et al. The Masaoka-Koga stage classification for thymic malignancies: clarification and definition of terms. J Thorac Oncol 2011;6(7 Suppl 3):S1710–6.

15. Edge SB, Edge SB, American Joint Committee on C. AJCC cancer staging manual. 8th edition. New York (NY): Springer.; 2017.

16. Nicholson AG, Detterbeck FC, Marino M, et al. The IASLC/ITMIG thymic epithelial tumors staging project: proposals for the T component for the forthcoming (8th) edition of the TNM classification of malignant tumors. J Thorac Oncol 2014;9(9 Suppl 2):S73–80.

17. Bhora FY, Chen DJ, Detterbeck FC, et al. The ITMIG/IASLC Thymic epithelial tumors staging project: a proposed lymph node map for thymic epithelial tumors in the forthcoming 8th edition of the TNM classification of malignant tumors. J Thorac Oncol 2014;9(9 Suppl 2):S88–96.

18. Kondo K, Van Schil P, Detterbeck FC, et al. The IASLC/ITMIG Thymic Epithelial Tumors Staging Project: proposals for the N and M components for the forthcoming (8th) edition of the TNM classification of malignant tumors. J Thorac Oncol 2014;9(9 Suppl 2):S81–7.

19. Travis WD, Brambilla E, Nicholson AG, et al. The 2015 World Health Organization classification of lung tumors: impact of genetic, clinical and radiologic advances since the 2004 classification. J Thorac Oncol 2015;10(9):1243–60.

20. Marx A, Chan JK, Coindre JM, et al. The 2015 World Health Organization classification of tumors of the thymus: continuity and changes. J Thorac Oncol 2015;10(10):1383–95.

21. Roden AC. Evolution of classification of thymic epithelial tumors in the era of Dr Thomas V. Colby. Arch Pathol Lab Med 2017;141(2):232–46.

22. Detterbeck FC, Moran C, Huang J, et al. Which way is up? Policies and procedures for surgeons and pathologists regarding resection specimens of thymic malignancy. J Thorac Oncol 2011;6(7 Suppl 3): S1730–8.

23. Weissferdt A, Moran CA. The impact of neoadjuvant chemotherapy on the histopathological assessment of thymomas: a clinicopathological correlation of 28 cases treated with a similar regimen. Lung 2013;191(4):379–83.

24. Nishino M, Ashiku SK, Kocher ON, et al. The thymus: a comprehensive review. Radiographics 2006;26(2): 335–48.

25. Carter BW, Benveniste MF, Madan R, et al. ITMIG classification of mediastinal compartments and multidisciplinary approach to mediastinal masses. Radiographics 2017;37(2):413–36.

26. Carter BW, Tomiyama N, Bhora FY, et al. A modern definition of mediastinal compartments. J Thorac Oncol 2014;9(9 Suppl 2):S97–101.

27. Araki T, Nishino M, Gao W, et al. Normal thymus in adults: appearance on CT and associations with age, sex, BMI and smoking. Eur Radiol 2016;26(1): 15–24.

28. Ackman JB, Kovacina B, Carter BW, et al. Sex difference in normal thymic appearance in adults 20-30 years of age. Radiology 2013;268(1):245–53.

29. Benveniste MF, Rosado-de-Christenson ML, Sabloff BS, et al. Role of imaging in the diagnosis, staging, and treatment of thymoma. Radiographics 2011;31(7):1847–61 [discussion 1861-1843].

30. Marom EM, Milito MA, Moran CA, et al. Computed tomography findings predicting invasiveness of thymoma. J Thorac Oncol 2011;6(7):1274–81.

31. Rosado-de-Christenson ML, Galobardes J, Moran CA. Thymoma: radiologic-pathologic correlation. Radiographics 1992;12(1):151–68.

32. McInnis MC, Flores EJ, Shepard JA, et al. Pitfalls in the imaging and interpretation of benign thymic lesions: how thymic MRI can help. AJR Am J Roentgenol 2016;206(1):W1–8.

33. Priola AM, Priola SM, Ciccone G, et al. Differentiation of rebound and lymphoid thymic hyperplasia from anterior mediastinal tumors with dual-echo chemical-shift MR imaging in adulthood: reliability of the chemical-shift ratio and signal intensity index. Radiology 2015;274(1):238–49.

34. Marom EM. Advances in thymoma imaging. J Thorac Imaging 2013;28(2):69–80. quiz 81-63.

35. Carter BW, Lichtenberger JP 3rd, Benveniste MF. MR imaging of thymic epithelial neoplasms. Top Magn Reson Imaging 2018;27(2):65–71.

36. Broncano J, Alvarado-Benavides AM, Bhalla S, et al. Role of advanced magnetic resonance imaging in the assessment of malignancies of the mediastinum. World J Radiol 2019;11(3):27–45.

37. Benveniste MF, Moran CA, Mawlawi O, et al. FDG PET-CT aids in the preoperative assessment of patients with newly diagnosed thymic epithelial malignancies. J Thorac Oncol 2013;8(4):502–10.

38. den Bakker MA, Roden AC, Marx A, et al. Histologic classification of thymoma: a practical guide for routine cases. J Thorac Oncol 2014;9(9 Suppl 2): S125–30.

39. Detterbeck FC, Stratton K, Giroux D, et al. The IASLC/ITMIG thymic epithelial tumors staging project: proposal for an evidence-based stage classification system for the forthcoming (8th) edition of the TNM classification of malignant tumors. J Thorac Oncol 2014;9(9 Suppl 2):S65–72.

40. Park S, Park IK, Kim YT, et al. Comparison of neoadjuvant chemotherapy followed by surgery to upfront surgery for thymic malignancy. Ann Thorac Surg 2019;107(2):355–62.

41. Nasseri F, Eftekhari F. Clinical and radiologic review of the normal and abnormal thymus: pearls and pitfalls. Radiographics 2010;30(2):413–28.

42. Tseng Y-L. Thymic carcinoma: a rare cancer requiring special attention. Formos J Surg 2011; 44(4):136–40.

43. Marx A, Strobel P, Badve SS, et al. ITMIG consensus statement on the use of the WHO histological classification of thymoma and thymic carcinoma: refined definitions, histological criteria, and reporting. J Thorac Oncol 2014;9(5):596–611.

44. Li HR, Gao J, Jin C, et al. Comparison between CT and MRI in the diagnostic accuracy of thymic masses. J Cancer 2019;10(14):3208–13.

45. Harris K, Elsayegh D, Azab B, et al. Thymoma calcification: is it clinically meaningful? World J Surg Oncol 2011;9:95.

46. Ackman JB, Wu CC. MRI of the thymus. AJR Am J Roentgenol 2011;197(1):W15–20.

47. Sasaki M, Kuwabara Y, Ichiya Y, et al. Differential diagnosis of thymic tumors using a combination of 11C-methionine PET and FDG PET. J Nucl Med 1999;40(10):1595–601.

48. Nakagawa K, Takahashi S, Endo M, et al. Can (18)F-FDG PET predict the grade of malignancy in thymic epithelial tumors? An evaluation of only resected tumors. Cancer Manag Res 2017;9:761–8.

49. Drevet G, Collaud S, Tronc F, et al. Optimal management of thymic malignancies: current perspectives. Cancer Manag Res 2019;11:6803–14.

50. Shimamoto A, Ashizawa K, Kido Y, et al. CT and MRI findings of thymic carcinoid. Br J Radiol 2017; 90(1071):20150341.

51. Bohnenberger H, Dinter H, Konig A, et al. Neuroendocrine tumors of the thymus and mediastinum. J Thorac Dis 2017;9(Suppl 15):S1448–57.

52. Fukai I, Masaoka A, Fujii Y, et al. Thymic neuroendocrine tumor (thymic carcinoid): a clinicopathologic study in 15 patients. Ann Thorac Surg 1999;67(1): 208–11.

53. Carrasquillo JA, Chen CC. Molecular imaging of neuroendocrine tumors. Semin Oncol 2010;37(6): 662–79.

54. Girard N. Neuroendocrine tumors of the thymus: the oncologist point of view. J Thorac Dis 2017;9(Suppl 15):S1491–500.

55. Fallahi B, Manafi-Farid R, Eftekhari M, et al. Diagnostic efficiency of (68)Ga-DOTATATE PET/CT as compared to (99m)Tc-Octreotide SPECT/CT and conventional morphologic modalities in neuroendocrine tumors. Asia Ocean J Nucl Med Biol 2019; 7(2):129–40.

56. Maxwell JE, Howe JR. Imaging in neuroendocrine tumors: an update for the clinician. Int J Endocr Oncol 2015;2(2):159–68.

57. Ma K, Liu Y, Xue Z, et al. Treatment, prognostic markers, and survival in thymic neuroendocrine tumors: a single center experience of 41 patients. Medicine (Baltimore) 2017;96(43):e7842.

# Thymic Epithelial Neoplasms
## Tumor-Node-Metastasis Staging

Marcelo F.K. Benveniste, MD[a],*, Sonia L. Betancourt Cuellar, MD[a],
Brett W. Carter, MD[b], Chad D. Strange, MD[a], Edith M. Marom, MD[c]

## KEYWORDS

- Thymic epithelial neoplasms • Thymoma • Thymic carcinoma • Thymic neuroendocrine tumors
- TNM • Staging

## KEY POINTS

- Despite sharing a standardized staging system and many imaging characteristics, thymic epithelial neoplasms, including thymoma, thymic carcinoma, and thymic neuroendocrine tumors, differ from each other in several key clinical characteristics.
- The tumor-node-metastasis (TNM) staging system developed for thymic epithelial neoplasms correlates with patient survival and outcomes.
- The individual TNM descriptors are organized into specific stage groups.
- As part of the International Association for the study of Lung Cancer/International Thymic Malignancy Interest Group staging project, a lymph node map was developed that is similar to those developed for other neoplasms such as lung cancer.
- Although computed tomography (CT) is the imaging modality of choice for assessing the primary tumor and determining the T stage, MR imaging may be used to help assess for local invasion, and fluorodeoxyglucose PET/CT can be useful in identifying involved lymph nodes and metastases that may be overlooked on CT.

## INTRODUCTION

Thymic epithelial neoplasms, a group of tumors including thymoma, thymic carcinoma, and thymic neuroendocrine cancers, are the most common primary malignancies of the prevascular mediastinum.[1] As surgical resection is the cornerstone of treatment, accurate staging is necessary to differentiate between patients who are operative candidates and those who are not.[2] Numerous staging systems have been developed over the years; however, their interpretation and implementation has been nonuniform. A partnership between the International Association for the study of Lung Cancer (IASLC) and the International Thymic Malignancy Interest Group (ITMIG) recently resulted in the creation of the first tumor-node-metastasis (TNM) staging system, which was adopted by the Union Internationale Contre le Cancer (UICC) and the American Joint Commission on Cancer (AJCC),[3–5] effectively replacing previous staging schemes in January 2017.[6] The objective of this article is to review the TNM staging system developed for thymic epithelial neoplasms and the role of imaging.

## GENERAL CONSIDERATIONS

Despite sharing the same staging system and many imaging characteristics, thymoma, thymic carcinoma, and carcinoid tumors differ from each other in several key clinical characteristics.

[a] Division of Diagnostic Imaging, MD Anderson Cancer Center, 1515 Holcombe Boulevard, Unit 1478, Houston, TX 77030, USA; [b] Department of Thoracic Imaging, MD Anderson Cancer Center, 1515 Holcombe Boulevard, Unit 1478, Houston, TX 77030, USA; [c] Department of Diagnostic Radiology, The Chaim Sheba Medical Center, Affiliated with the Tel Aviv University, Tel Aviv, 2 Derech Sheba, Ramat Gan 5265601, Israel
* Corresponding author. Department of Thoracic Radiology, The University of Texas MD Anderson Cancer Center, Unit 1478, 1515 Holcombe Boulevard, Houston, TX 77030.
E-mail address: mfbenveniste@mdanderson.org

Radiol Clin N Am 59 (2021) 183–192
https://doi.org/10.1016/j.rcl.2020.11.006
0033-8389/21/© 2020 Elsevier Inc. All rights reserved.

Thymoma, the most common thymic epithelial neoplasm, typically occurs in patients older than 40 years, peaking in the seventh decade, and affects men and women equally.[1,7] Most thymomas are solid neoplasms that are localized to the thymus but may exhibit aggressive behavior such as invasion of adjacent structures. Although involvement of the pleura and pericardium may occur, distant metastases are rare. With the widespread availability and increased use of computed tomography (CT), a greater number of thymomas are incidentally discovered while patients are asymptomatic. When patients present with clinical symptoms, such as dysphagia, diaphragm paralysis, or superior vena cava syndrome, these are usually related to local effects from compression or invasion of adjacent structures.[8] Other patients may present with paraneoplastic syndromes, the most common of which is myasthenia gravis. Between 30% and 50% of patients with thymoma have myasthenia gravis, whereas only 10% to 15% of patients with myasthenia gravis have a thymoma.[9] Additional paraneoplastic syndromes such as hypogammaglobulinemia and pure red cell aplasia are seen in 10% and 5% of patients with thymoma, respectively.[10] Thymoma has also been associated with autoimmune disorders such as systemic lupus erythematosus, polymyositis, and myocarditis.[11]

Thymic carcinoma comprises 20% of thymic epithelial neoplasms, with a mean age of 50 years at presentation.[12,13] It is more aggressive than thymoma and is more likely to result in local invasion and intrathoracic lymphadenopathy. At presentation, 50% to 65% of patients have distant metastases.[14,15] Symptoms usually relate to the intrathoracic local effects of the neoplasm, principally compression, and invasion of adjacent structures. In contrast to thymoma, paraneoplastic syndromes rarely accompany thymic carcinoma.

Thymic neuroendocrine neoplasms comprise only 2% to 5% of thymic epithelial neoplasms, most of which are carcinoid tumors.[16] Thymic neuroendocrine tumors are more frequent in men, typically occurring in the fourth and fifth decades of life.[17] Clinical symptoms reported by patients and imaging findings on cross-sectional imaging are similar to those encountered in thymic carcinoma.[18] One-third of patients are asymptomatic, and the tumor may be discovered when imaging is performed as routine surveillance of patients with multiple endocrine neoplasia type 1, as they are predisposed to develop thymic carcinoids.[16] Acromegaly, syndrome of inappropriate secretion of antidiuretic hormone, and carcinoid syndrome, although rare, are paraneoplastic syndromes associated with thymic neuroendocrine tumors.[19,20]

## PROGNOSTICATION

Multiple key pieces of information related to thymic epithelial neoplasms affect patient prognosis, including anatomic spread of disease, histologic classification, age, and functional status. The histologic classification of thymic epithelial neoplasms was most recently updated by the World Health Organization (WHO) Consensus Committee in 2015.[21] Thymomas are classified into 5 separate histologic subtypes—A, AB, B1, B2, B3—based on the morphology of the neoplastic epithelial cells together with the lymphocyte. Thymic carcinomas are divided into multiple histologic subtypes including adenocarcinoma, squamous, basaloid, mucoepidermoid, lymphoepithelioma-like, clear cell, and sarcomatoid carcinomas. Thymic neuroendocrine tumors are divided into carcinoid, large cell carcinomas, and small cell carcinomas. Although thymic carcinoma and thymic neuroendocrine neoplasms are associated with a poorer prognosis compared with thymoma, the different subtypes of thymoma have little practical clinical use. The WHO histologic classification lacks inter- and intraobserver reproducibility and clinical predictive value.[22,23] In addition, multiple WHO subtypes are often present in the same tumor, which makes classification more challenging especially in needle biopsy specimen where the predominant tumor subtype may not be sampled.[23] Management decisions rest primarily on the stage of disease and the completeness of resection, both of which were repeatedly found to correlate with prognosis.[24–26]

Multiple anatomic staging schemes have been used over the years, all based on small series from single institutions.[27] Before 2017, the most widely used staging systems included the Masaoka system, proposed in 1981, based on 91 patients,[28] or and its variant, the Masaoka-Koga system, proposed in 1994, based on 79 patients.[29] The Masaoka-Koga staging is based on the gross and microscopic properties of the tumor. Stage I tumors are characterized by complete encapsulation; stage II by microscopic invasion through the capsule (IIa) or macroscopic invasion into surrounding fat (IIb); stage III by invasion into any neighboring organs such as the pericardium, great vessels, trachea, esophagus, or lung; and stage IV by pleural or pericardial metastases (IVa) or hematogenous or lymphatic metastases (IVb).

Several limitations of the Masaoka-based staging systems have been described. The reliance on a capsule for staging was difficult, as not all thymomas have a complete capsule. Masaoka stage III included involvement of many organs; however, the staging was based on such a small number of patients that there was insufficient power to address the nuances of the stage. The TNM staging system developed by the IASLC and ITMIG used a retrospective database of 10,808 cases gathered from 105 institutions worldwide, which correlates with overall survival.[30]

## TUMOR-NECROSIS-METASTASIS DESCRIPTORS
### Primary Tumor

The tumor (T) descriptor is determined by the presence and extent of local tumor invasion[5] (Table 1). T1 describes encapsulated or unencapsulated tumors with or without extension into the adjacent prevascular (perithymic) mediastinal fat. The T1 category is further divided into T1a with no mediastinal pleural involvement or T1b with direct invasion of the mediastinal pleura (Fig. 1). T2 describes lesions with direct invasion of the pericardium (Fig. 2). T3 is characterized by tumor involvement of the lung, brachiocephalic vein, superior vena cava, phrenic nerve, chest wall, or extrapericardial pulmonary artery or veins (Fig. 3). Finally, T4 tumors include those that invade the aorta (ascending, arch, or descending), aortic arch vessels (brachiocephalic, carotid, and subclavian arteries), intrapericardial pulmonary artery, myocardium, trachea, or the esophagus (Fig. 4).

### Regional Lymph Nodes

The lymph node (N) descriptor is determined by the presence or absence of intrathoracic lymph node involvement. *The N stage defines lymph node regions as defined by the IASLC/ITMIG project*[31] *(KP).* N0 describes the absence of lymph node metastasis. N1 and N2 represent involved lymph nodes located in the prevascular and deep spaces of the mediastinum, respectively, as outlined in the specific lymph node map created for use with thymic epithelial neoplasms (Fig. 5). N1 node includes prevascular mediastinal and perithymic lymph nodes, and N2 disease describes deep intrathoracic and cervical lymph nodes, including tracheobronchial and aortopulmonary window, internal mammary, deep cervical, and supraclavicular lymph nodes (see Table 1).

### Distant Metastases

The metastasis (M) descriptor is divided into 3 categories based on the presence and location of metastatic disease (see Table 1). M0 indicates the absence of metastasis. The M1 descriptor is subdivided into 2 components—M1a and M1b—and reflects whether pleural and pericardial nodules (M1a) (Fig. 6) or distant organ metastases (M1b), including pulmonary intraparenchymal metastatic nodules and extrathoracic (distant) metastases, are present (Fig. 7).

### Stage Groups

*The individual TNM descriptors are organized into specific stage groups (KP)* (Fig. 8). The definitions of stages I, II, IIIA, and IIIB are based on the T category in the absence of lymph node involvement (N0) and the absence of metastases (M0). In addition, the M stage separates pleural or pericardial

| Table 1 Tumor staging | | |
|---|---|---|
| T | T1a | Encapsulated or unencapsulated, with or without extension into mediastinal fat |
| | T1b | Extension into mediastinal pleura |
| | T2 | Involvement of pericardium |
| | T3 | Involvement of lung, brachiocephalic vein, superior vena cava, chest wall, phrenic nerve, hilar (extrapericardial) pulmonary vessels |
| | T4 | Involvement of aorta, arch vessels, main pulmonary artery, myocardium, trachea, or esophagus |
| N | N0 | No lymph node metastasis |
| | N1 | Involvement of anterior (perithymic) lymph nodes |
| | N2 | Involvement of deep intrathoracic or cervical lymph nodes |
| M | M0 | No metastasis |
| | M1a | Pleural or pericardial metastatic nodules |
| | M1b | Pulmonary intraparenchymal metastatic nodule or distant organ metastasis |

From Detterbeck, F.C., et al., The IASLC/ITMIG Thymic Epithelial Tumors Staging Project: proposal for an evidence-based stage classification system for the forthcoming (8th) edition of the TNM classification of malignant tumors. J Thorac Oncol, 2014. 9(9 Suppl 2): p. S65-72; with permission.

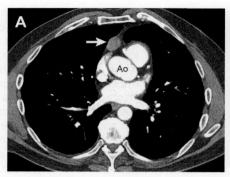
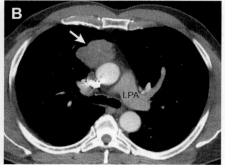

Fig. 1. T1 tumors. (*A*) Contrast-enhanced axial CT of the chest at the level of the ascending aorta (Ao) shows a 3-cm oval mass in the right prevascular mediastinum (*arrow*) surrounded by fat. A thymoma with no capsular invasion was diagnosed at surgery, representing T1a disease. (*B*) Contrast-enhanced axial CT of the chest at the level of the left pulmonary artery (LPA) shows a 6-cm thymoma abutting the ascending aorta with a lobular contour with the lung (*arrow*). At surgery there was tumor invasion into perithymic adipose tissue and pleura only. Abutment of structures, such as the aorta or lung, does not necessarily translate to invasion.

nodules (M1a) from pulmonary nodules or distant metastases (M1b). In contrast, stages IVA and IVB are determined by the N or M categories, regardless of the T descriptor (see **Fig. 8**).

## LIMITATIONS OF THE TUMOR-NECROSIS-METASTASIS STAGING SYSTEM

Although the newly developed TNM staging system for thymic epithelial neoplasms described herein enables more detailed prognostication based on anatomic tumor spread, a few notable limitations have been described. Because most of the collected data were based on surgical cases, advanced disease is underrepresented when compared with earlier stage thymic epithelial neoplasms.[3] Tumor size, a quantitative parameter that can be easily be assessed, is used in staging other intrathoracic malignancies and is not part of the TNM staging system, as it did not correlate with advanced disease or overall survival and did not predict the ability to perform complete tumor resection.[5,32] Despite the size of the dataset used to develop the TNM staging system, a limited number of cases with T4 disease prevented a detailed assessment of behavior based on involvement of different organs within a specific histologic type of neoplasm. In addition, the small number of thymic neuroendocrine neoplasms limited a separate analysis of T categories in this tumor type.[3]

## TREATMENT

Treatment of thymic epithelial neoplasms is based on staging, although there are no standardized guidelines concerning optimal management.[33] The main role of clinical staging is to distinguish between early disease (stage I) and advanced

disease (stages II–IV), identifying candidates that may benefit from preoperative neoadjuvant therapy. A multidisciplinary approach should be developed before treatment decisions are made, including involvement of thoracic surgeons, medical oncologists, radiation oncologists, and diagnostic radiologists. Surgical resection is the cornerstone of treatment of thymic epithelial neoplasms.[2] The goal is complete resection, even in advanced stages when neighboring organs are involved, as it improves survival and has been shown to be the most important predictor of outcomes.[2,34,35] There is general agreement that early stage disease is treated with surgical resection. With incomplete surgical resection confirmed by microscopic disease at the surgical site, multimodality therapy, including chemotherapy and postoperative radiotherapy, is recommended to

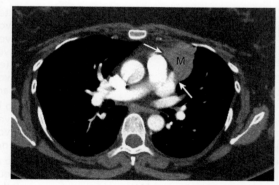

Fig. 2. T2 tumor. Contrast-enhanced axial CT of the chest demonstrates a 4-cm mass (M) abutting the pericardium (*arrows*). At surgery, a thymic carcinoma involving the perithymic adipose tissue and pericardium was detected, consistent with a T2 tumor.

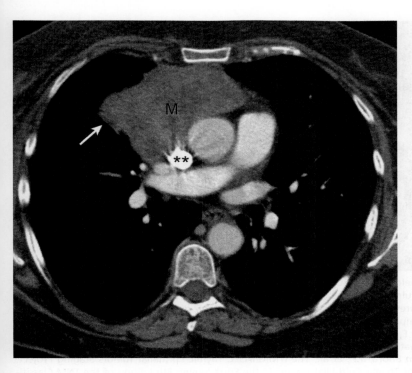

Fig. 3. T3 tumor. Contrast-enhanced axial CT of the chest demonstrates a prevascular mediastinal mass (M), which forms a lobular border with the lung (*arrow*) and surrounds a portion of the superior vena cava (*double asterisk*). At surgery, a thymoma was diagnosed and involvement of the lung and superior vena cava was confirmed, the findings of which are consistent with T3 disease.

achieve complete disease eradication.[33,36,37] Neoadjuvant chemotherapy is recommended for potentially resectable locally advanced thymic malignancies.[38,39] Following surgical resection, postoperative radiation therapy is recommended, as these patients are at higher risk of recurrence.[40] Solitary metastasis and ipsilateral pleural metastatic disease are managed surgically combined with chemoradiotherapy. Patients with extrathoracic metastases are treated with chemotherapy with palliative intent.

## THE ROLE OF IMAGING AND ITS LIMITATIONS

Although staging is determined by histologic examination of the resected tumor, initial treatment decisions are imaging based, determining those patients that receive upfront surgery, neoadjuvant therapy followed by surgery, and those who are not surgical candidates. Thus, the role of the radiologist is to identify local tumor invasion and spread of tumor to mediastinal lymph nodes, pleura, pericardium, and distant organs.

### Chest Radiography

The role of chest radiography in clinical staging is limited, although findings that suggest locally advanced disease, including irregular borders of the mediastinal mass and elevation of the hemidiaphragm related to phrenic nerve involvement, may be ascertained.

### Computed Tomography

CT is the imaging modality of choice for staging thymic epithelial neoplasms, as it provides excellent spatial resolution for identifying local invasion. The use of intravenous iodinated contrast material

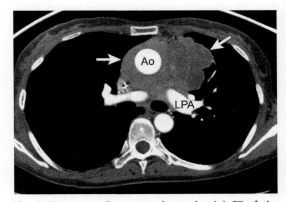

Fig. 4. T4 tumor. Contrast-enhanced axial CT of the chest shows a large prevascular mediastinal mass (*arrows*) encircling the ascending aorta (Ao) and left pulmonary artery (LPA). At surgery, this thymoma involved the mediastinal pleura, lung parenchyma, pericardium, aorta, and left pulmonary artery, consistent with a T4 tumor.

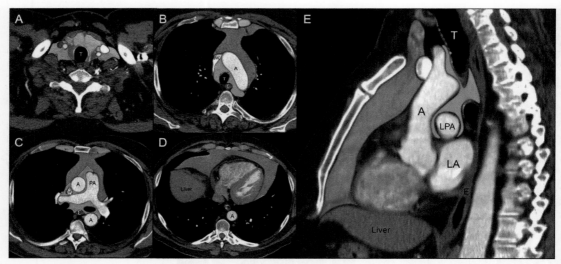

**Fig. 5.** The lymph node map developed by IASLC and ITMIG. (*A*) Axial CT images (*A–D*) at the level of the thoracic inlet (*A*), transverse aorta (*B*), pulmonary artery (*C*), and base of the heart (*D*) show N1 lymph nodes (*orange*), including anterior cervical and prevascular mediastinal lymph nodes, and N2 disease (*green*), including deep cervical and visceral mediastinal lymph nodes. Sagittal CT images (*E*) demonstrate N1 lymph nodes (*orange*) and N2 lymph nodes (*green*). T, trachea; E, esophagus; A, aorta; SVC, superior vena cava; PA, pulmonary artery; LPA, left pulmonary artery; ITMIG, International Thymic Malignancy Interest Group; IASCL, International Association for the Study of Lung Cancer. (*From* Bhora, Y.F., et al., The ITMIG/IASLC Thymic Epithelial Tumors Staging Project: A Proposed Lymph Node Map for Thymic Epithelial Tumors in the Forthcoming 8th Edition of the TNM Classification of Malignant Tumors. Journal of Thoracic Oncology, 2014. 9(9 Suppl 2): p. S88-S96; with permission.)

is indicated for this purpose. Direct signs of invasion include endoluminal soft tissue, irregularity of the vessel lumen, and vascular encasement or obliteration. Although the assessment of tumor extension into the lung by CT is limited, findings such as a lobular lung-tumor border are suggestive. However, confirmation of this extent of invasion is usually delineated at surgery. The role of CT in differentiating tumor abutment from involvement of adjacent structures is also limited. Prior studies have demonstrated that detection of tumor abutting greater than or equal to 50% of a vessel circumference correlates with advanced disease (Masaoka-Koga stage III–IV) and is a potential predictor of an incomplete tumor surgical resection.[41,42] *When assessing the N and M descriptors, CT has a high sensitivity for detecting lesions suspicious for metastatic disease (KP).* Involvement of cardiac structures such as the epicardial fat and pericardium may be identifiable on CT (**Fig. 9**). Pericardial effusion may suggest cardiac metastasis although tumors invading the pericardium may cause an inflammatory reaction with consequent effusion as well.[43]

### MR Imaging

MR imaging is typically used as a problem-solving tool for staging questions arising from CT imaging or is reserved for assessing patients with a contraindication to intravenous iodinated contrast material.[32] MR imaging is characterized by superior contrast resolution related to CT and may be used to better define local invasion but also has the ability to image in motion for the assessment of adherence/invasion and functionality of the phrenic nerve when there is concern for invasion. Fat-suppression techniques may be useful in differentiating tumor involvement from

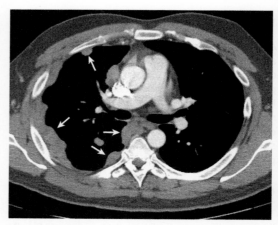

**Fig. 6.** M1a disease. Contrast-enhanced axial CT of the chest shows multiple right pleural metastases (*arrows*) from a thymoma (not shown).

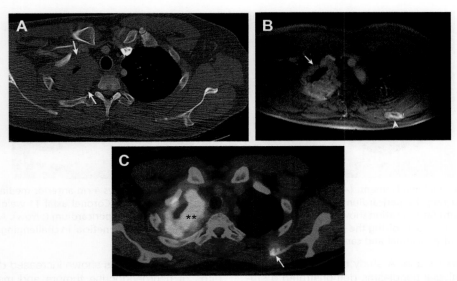

**Fig. 7.** M1b disease. (*A*) Contrast-enhanced axial CT of the chest demonstrates concentric right pleural nodular thickening (*arrows*) consistent with pleural metastatic disease from thymic carcinoma (not shown). (*B*) Axial T1-weighted fast spin echo with fat saturation MR image after the administration of paramagnetic intravenous contrast, performed 3 days following the CT, shows the right circumferential pleural metastatic disease (*arrow*) and an enhancing left scapular metastasis (*arrow head*). With its superior contrast resolution, MR imaging is a valuable tool in the assessment of the chest wall and soft tissues and in identifying distant metastatic disease that may be overlooked on CT. (*C*) Fused axial FDG PET/CT shows marked FDG uptake in the metastases to the pleura (*double asterisk*) and scapula (*arrow*), typical of thymic carcinoma.

surrounding fat. Cardiac MR imaging is the optimal imaging modality for evaluating suspected or known involvement of the heart and/or pericardium (see **Fig. 9**). In addition, MR imaging is considered superior to CT in identifying chest wall invasion and may result in improved visualization of soft tissue metastases previously undetected on CT (see **Fig. 7**B).[44] A study comparing tumor stage according to IASCL/ITMIG classification in 64 patients with thymic epithelial neoplasms showed that the staging capabilities of MR imaging were superior compared with CT.[45] There is controversy regarding the ability of apparent diffusion coefficient (ADC) values to

| PRIMARY TUMOR (T) | | | | | | |
|---|---|---|---|---|---|---|
| | | **T1** | **T2** | **T3** | **T4** | |
| | **N0** | I | II | IIIA | IIIB | **M0** |
| | **N1** | | IVA | | | |
| **LYMPH NODES (N)** | **N0, N1** | | IVA | | | **M1a** |
| | **N2** | | IVB | | | **M0, M1a** |
| | **Any N** | | IVB | | | **M1b** |

(rightmost column label, vertical: **METASTASIS (M)**)

**Fig. 8.** Tumor stage groups.

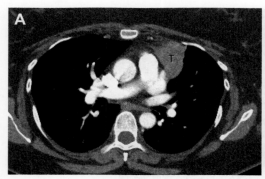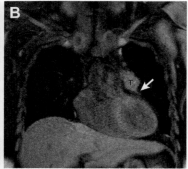

**Fig. 9.** Pericardial Involvement. (*A*) Contrast-enhanced chest CT scan demonstrates 4 cm anterior mediastinal tumor (T) abutting the pericardium with no obvious pericardial involvement. (*B*) Coronal axial T1-weighted fast spin echo with fat saturation shows the tumor (T) with extends into the adjacent pericardium (*arrow*). At surgery a thymic carcinoma involving the pericardium was detected. MRI of the chest is beneficial in challenging cases for assessment of pericardial and cardiac involvement.

predict tumor stage. A study of 30 patients with thymic epithelial neoplasms demonstrated a statistically significant difference in ADC values for early stage versus advanced stage disease,[46] although a different analysis of 41 patients evaluated with MR imaging showed that ADC values could not discriminate early from advanced disease.[47]

### Nuclear Medicine

In general, fluorodeoxyglucose (FDG) PET/CT does not have a routine role in staging of thymoma. In a study assessing 51 patients with thymic epithelial neoplasms, there was no association between higher FDG uptake and advanced disease.[48]

FDG PET/CT has no role in T-staging due to its poor spatial resolution. However, as with other malignancies, FDG PET/CT is particularly useful for determining the N and M descriptors and sometimes identifying findings overlooked by CT (see **Fig. 7**C). Unfortunately, there are thymomas that are not FDG-avid, and thus, for them, FDG PET/CT is not useful. However, because thymic carcinoma has high FDG uptake and has a tendency to present at advanced stage, FDG PET/CT may play an important role for the assessment of these tumors. For example, a study assessing FDG PET/CT in 33 patients with thymic carcinoma demonstrated benefit by enabling detection of lymph node and distant metastases originally overlooked by CT.[49]

[68]Ga-labeled somatostatin analogues, including [68]Ga-DOTATATE or [68]Ga-DOTA-try-octreotide (DOTATOC), have replaced imaging with Indium[111] Octreotide. As PET radiotracers, they provide improved spatial resolution for disease detection as compared with Indium[111] Octreotide.[50] Preoperative [68]Ga-DOTA-somatostatin

analogue-PET/CT has shown increased detection rates of neuroendocrine tumors and may serve as an additional tool for assessment of disease spread in thymic epithelial neoplasms.[51,52] However, imaging with somatostatin analogues is usually reserved for selection of candidates for second-line chemotherapy with somatostatin analogues.

### SUMMARY

The TNM staging system for thymic epithelial neoplasms is inconclusive of all malignant tumors classified as such, is universally accepted, and correlates with survival. Imaging enables accurate staging of patients and determination of effective treatment strategies. Thus, radiologists should be familiar with this system to correctly differentiate between patients who may benefit from upfront surgery and those who require neoadjuvant therapy.

### CLINICS CARE POINTS

- To understand different staging systems for thymic malignancies and implications in prognosis and treatment.
- To identify role of imaging modalities and its limitations in the TNM staging of thymic malignancies.

### ACKNOWLEDGMENTS

The authors thank Kelly Kage for creating the drawings in **Table 1** and **Figs. 5** and **8**.

### DISCLOSURE

Financial disclosures: B.W.Carter: Royalties from Elsevier. E.M. Marom: Honorarium for lectures: Bristol-Myers Squibb, Boehringer Ingelheim,

Merck Sharp & Dohme. Chief Medical Officer: Voxellence. Additional co-authors have no financial disclosures.

## REFERENCES

1. Morgenthaler TI, Brown LR, Colby TV, et al. Thymoma. Mayo Clin Proc 1993;68(11):1110–23.
2. Girard N, Mornex F, Van Houtte P, et al. Thymoma: a focus on current therapeutic management. J Thorac Oncol 2009;4(1):119–26.
3. Detterbeck FC, Stratton K, Giroux D, et al. The IASLC/ITMIG Thymic Epithelial Tumors Staging Project: proposal for an evidence-based stage classification system for the forthcoming (8th) edition of the TNM classification of malignant tumors. J Thorac Oncol 2014;9(9 Suppl 2):S65–72.
4. Kondo K, Van Schil P, Detterbeck FC, et al. The IASLC/ITMIG Thymic Epithelial Tumors Staging Project: proposals for the N and M components for the forthcoming (8th) edition of the TNM classification of malignant tumors. J Thorac Oncol 2014;9(9 Suppl 2):S81–7.
5. Nicholson AG, Detterbeck FC, Marino M, et al. The IASLC/ITMIG Thymic Epithelial Tumors Staging Project: proposals for the T Component for the forthcoming (8th) edition of the TNM classification of malignant tumors. J Thorac Oncol 2014;9(9 Suppl 2):S73–80.
6. Ruffini E, Wentao F, Francesco G, et al. The international association for the study of lung cancer thymic tumors staging project: the impact of the eighth edition of the Union for International Cancer Control and American Joint Committee on Cancer TNM stage classification of thymic tumors. J Thorac Oncol 2019;15(3):436–47.
7. Engels EA. Epidemiology of thymoma and associated malignancies. J Thorac Oncol 2010;5(10 Suppl 4):S260–5.
8. Lewis JE, Wick MR, Scheithauer BW, et al. Thymoma. A clinicopathologic review. Cancer 1987;60(11):2727–43.
9. Osserman KE, Genkins G. Studies in myasthenia gravis: review of a twenty-year experience in over 1200 patients. Mt Sinai J Med 1971;38(6):497–537.
10. Cameron RB, Loehrer P, Lee PP. Neoplasms of the mediastinum. DeVita, Hellman, and Rosenberg's cancer: principles & practice of Oncology. 10th edition. Netherlands: Wolters Kluwer Health Adis (ESP); 2015.
11. Levy Y, Afek A, Sherer Y, et al. Malignant thymoma associated with autoimmune diseases: a retrospective study and review of the literature. Semin Arthritis Rheum 1998;28(2):73–9.
12. Nasseri F, Eftekhari F. Clinical and radiologic review of the normal and abnormal thymus: pearls and pitfalls. Radiographics 2010;30(2):413–28.
13. Webb WR, Higgins CB. Thoracic imaging : pulmonary and cardiovascular Radiology. Philadelphia: Wolters Kluwer Health; 2010.
14. Rosado-de-Christenson ML, Strollo DC, Marom EM. Imaging of thymic epithelial neoplasms. Hematol Oncol Clin North Am 2008;22(3):409–31.
15. Mittal MK, Sureka B, Sinha M, et al. Thymic masses: A radiological review. S Afr J Rad 2013;17(3):108–11.
16. Chaer R, Massad M, Evans A, et al. Primary neuroendocrine tumors of the thymus. Ann Thorac Surg 2002;74:1733–40.
17. Dusmet ME, McKneally MF. Pulmonary and thymic carcinoid tumors. World J Surg 1996;20(2):189–95.
18. McKneally CA, Suster S. Neuroendocrine carcinomas (carcinoid tumor) of the thymus. A clinicopathologic analysis of 80 cases. Am J Clin Pathol 2000;114(1):100–10.
19. Soga J, Yakuwa Y, Osaka M. Evaluation of 342 cases of mediastinal/thymic carcinoids collected from literature: a comparative study between typical carcinoids and atypical varieties. Ann Thorac Cardiovasc Surg 1999;5(5):285–92.
20. Jansson J, Svensson J, Bengtsson BA, et al. Acromegaly and Cushing's syndrome due to ectopic production of GHRH and ACTH by a thymic carcinoid tumour: in vitro responses to GHRH and GHRP-6. Clin Endocrinol (Oxf) 1998;48(2):243–50.
21. Marx A, Chan JK, Coindre JM, et al. The 2015 World Health Organization classification of tumors of the thymus: continuity and changes. J Thorac Oncol 2015;10(10):1383–95.
22. Rieker RJ, Hoegel J, Morresi-Hauf A, et al. Histologic classification of thymic epithelial tumors: Comparison of established classification schemes. Int J Cancer 2002;98(6):900–6.
23. Suster S, Moran CA. Histologic classification of thymoma: the World Health Organization and beyond. Hematol Oncol Clin North Am 2008;22(3):381–92.
24. Blumberg D, Port JL, Weksler B, et al. Thymoma: a multivariate analysis of factors predicting survival. Ann Thorac Surg 1995;60(4):908–14.
25. Nakagawa K, Asamura H, Matsuno Y, et al. Thymoma: a clinicopathologic study based on the new World Health Organization classification. J Thorac Cardiovasc Surg 2003;126(4):1134–40.
26. Wright CD, Wain JC, Wong DR, et al. Predictors of recurrence in thymic tumors: importance of invasion, World Health Organization histology, and size. J Thorac Cardiovasc Surg 2005;130(5):1413–21.
27. Filosso PL, Ruffini E, Lausi PO, et al. Historical perspectives: The evolution of the thymic epithelial tumors staging system. Lung Cancer 2014;83(2):126–32.
28. Masaoka A, Monden Y, Nakahara K, et al. Follow-up study of thymomas with special reference to their clinical stages. Cancer 1981;48(11):2485–92.

29. Koga K, Matsuno Y, Noguchi M, et al. A review of 79 thymomas: modification of staging system and reappraisal of conventional division into invasive and non-invasive thymoma. Pathol Int 1994;44(5): 359–67.

30. Detterbeck F. International thymic malignancies interest group: a way forward. J Thorac Oncol 2010; 5(10 Suppl 4):S365–70.

31. Bhora FY, Chen DJ, Detterbeck FC, et al. The ITMIG/IASLC thymic epithelial tumors staging project: a proposed lymph node map for thymic epithelial tumors in the forthcoming 8th edition of the TNM classification of malignant tumors. J Thorac Oncol 2014; 9(9 Suppl 2):S88–96.

32. Carter BW, Benveniste MF, Madan R, et al. IASLC/ITMIG staging system and lymph node map for thymic epithelial neoplasms. Radiographics 2017;37(3): 758.

33. Ruffini E, Van Raemdonck D, Detterbeck F, et al. Management of thymic tumors: a survey of current practice among members of the European Society of Thoracic Surgeons. J Thorac Oncol 2011;6(3): 614–23.

34. Elkiran ET, Abali H, Aksoy S, et al. Thymic epithelial neoplasia: a study of 58 cases. Med Oncol 2007; 24(2):197–201.

35. Ried M, Marx A, Götz A, et al. State of the art: diagnostic tools and innovative therapies for treatment of advanced thymoma and thymic carcinoma. Eur J Cardiothorac Surg 2016;49(6):1545–52.

36. National Comprehensive Cancer Network, NCCN Clinical Practice Guidelines in Oncology, Guidelines Version 1.2021, in Thymomas and Thymic Carcinomas. 2020. Available at: https://www.nccn.org.

37. Fuller CD, Ramahi EH, Aherne N, et al. Radiotherapy for thymic neoplasms. J Thorac Oncol 2010;5(10 Suppl 4):S327–35.

38. Park S, Park IK, Kim YT, et al. Comparison of neoadjuvant chemotherapy followed by surgery to upfront surgery for thymic malignancy. Ann Thorac Surg 2019;107(2):355–62.

39. Kanzaki R, Kanou T, Ose N, et al. Long-term outcomes of advanced thymoma in patients undergoing preoperative chemotherapy or chemoradiotherapy followed by surgery: a 20-year experience. Interact Cardiovasc Thorac Surg 2019; 28(3):360–7.

40. Lim YJ, Kim HJ, Wu HG. Role of postoperative radiotherapy in nonlocalized thymoma: propensity-matched analysis of surveillance, epidemiology, and end results database. J Thorac Oncol 2015; 10(9):1357–63.

41. Hayes SA, Huang J, Plodkowski AJ, et al. Preoperative computed tomography findings predict surgical resectability of thymoma. J Thorac Oncol 2014;9(7): 1023–30.

42. Marom EM, Milito MA, Moran CA, et al. Computed tomography findings predicting invasiveness of thymoma. J Thorac Oncol 2011;6(7):1274–81.

43. Lichtenberger JP 3rd, Reynolds DA, Keung J, et al. Metastasis to the heart: a radiologic approach to diagnosis with pathologic correlation. AJR Am J Roentgenol 2016;207(4):1–9.

44. Patz EF Jr, Shaffer K, Piwnica-Worms DR, et al. Malignant pleural mesothelioma: value of CT and MR imaging in predicting resectability. AJR Am J Roentgenol 1992;159(5):961–6.

45. Ohno Y, Kishida Y, Seki S, et al. Comparison of Interobserver Agreement and Diagnostic Accuracy for IASLC/ITMIG Thymic Epithelial Tumor Staging Among Co-registered FDG-PET/MRI, Whole-body MRI, Integrated FDG-PET/CT, and Conventional Imaging Examination with and without Contrast Media Administrations. Acad Radiol 2018. https://doi.org/10.1016/j.acra.2017.12.016.

46. Abdel Razek AA, Khairy M, Nada N. Diffusion-weighted MR imaging in thymic epithelial tumors: correlation with World Health Organization classification and clinical staging. Radiology 2014;273(1): 268–75.

47. Priola AM, Priola SM, Giraudo MT, et al. Diffusion-weighted magnetic resonance imaging of thymoma: ability of the Apparent Diffusion Coefficient in predicting the World Health Organization (WHO) classification and the Masaoka-Koga staging system and its prognostic significance on disease-free survival. Eur Radiol 2016;26(7):2126–38.

48. Benveniste MF, Moran CA, Mawlawi O, et al. FDG PET-CT aids in the preoperative assessment of patients with newly diagnosed thymic epithelial malignancies. J Thorac Oncol 2013;8(4):502–10.

49. Sung YM, Lee KS, Kim BT, et al. 18F-FDG PET/CT of thymic epithelial tumors: usefulness for distinguishing and staging tumor subgroups. J Nucl Med 2006;47(10):1628–34.

50. Buchmann I, Henze M, Engelbrecht S, et al. Comparison of 68Ga-DOTATOC PET and 111In-DTPAOC (Octreoscan) SPECT in patients with neuroendocrine tumours. Eur J Nucl Med Mol Imaging 2007; 34(10):1617–26.

51. Hephzibah J, Shanthly N, Oommen R. Diagnostic Utility of PET CT in Thymic Tumours with Emphasis on 68Ga-DOTATATE PET CT in Thymic Neuroendocrine Tumour - Experience at a Tertiary Level Hospital in India. J Clin Diagn Res 2014;8(9):QC01.

52. Norlen O, Montan H, Hellman P, et al. Preoperative (68)Ga-DOTA-Somatostatin Analog-PET/CT Hybrid Imaging Increases Detection Rate of Intra-abdominal Small Intestinal Neuroendocrine Tumor Lesions. World J Surg 2018;42(2):498–505.

# Imaging of the Middle and Visceral Mediastinum

Patrick P. Bourgouin, MD[a], Rachna Madan, MD[b],*

## KEYWORDS

- Visceral • Middle • Mediastinum • Lymphadenopathy • Foregut cyst • Paraganglioma

## KEY POINTS

- The middle or visceral mediastinum contains the heart, great vessels, lymph nodes, the esophagus and portions of the trachea.
- Computed tomography scanning is the primary imaging modality used to identify and characterize mediastinal abnormalities. MR imaging and nuclear medicine studies can help with problem solving and refining the differential diagnosis.
- Lymphadenopathy is the most common disease process involving the visceral mediastinum and occurs with a wide variety of benign and malignant processes.
- Other abnormalities that can be diagnosed on imaging include foregut duplication cysts, neoplasms and other lesions arising from the trachea and esophagus, and paragangliomas.
- In addition to identifying, localizing, and characterizing lesions in the visceral mediastinum, imaging plays an important role in directing invasive diagnostic procedures and monitoring response to treatment.

## INTRODUCTION

The middle or visceral mediastinum is notable for containing the heart, great vessels, lymph nodes, and portions of the esophagus and trachea. In terms of pathology, the most common abnormalities involving this compartment include lymphadenopathy, foregut duplication cysts such as bronchogenic and esophageal duplication cysts, tracheal and esophageal neoplasms, and other diseases. Imaging plays a key role in identifying and diagnosing these conditions as well as guiding biopsy or surgery if needed.

## NORMAL ANATOMY AND IMAGING TECHNIQUE

The mediastinum contains several vascular and nonvascular structures and its division into different compartments is crucial for localization and development of an accurate differential diagnosis. The International Thymic Malignancy Interest Group has developed a classification of mediastinal compartments based on cross-sectional imaging to help with characterization of mediastinal lesions and facilitate communication among medical specialties. This classification is accepted as a standard.[1,2]

The visceral mediastinal compartment is characterized by the following boundaries: (1) the thoracic inlet superiorly, (2) the diaphragm inferiorly, (3) the anterior aspect of the pericardium anteriorly, and (4) a vertical line situated 1 cm posterior to the anterior margin of each vertebral body posteriorly. Thus, it includes several important vascular structures such as the heart, thoracic aorta, intrapericardial pulmonary arteries, superior vena cava, and thoracic duct. Nonvascular structures incorporated in this compartment include portions of the trachea, including the carina, the esophagus, and the lymph nodes.[1,2]

[a] Department of Radiology, Brigham and Women's Hospital, 75 Francis Street, Boston, MA 02115, USA;
[b] Division of Thoracic Imaging, Department of Radiology, Brigham and Women's Hospital, Harvard Medical School, 75 Francis Street, Boston, MA 02115, USA
* Corresponding author.
*E-mail address:* rmadan@bwh.harvard.edu

Radiol Clin N Am 59 (2021) 193–204
https://doi.org/10.1016/j.rcl.2020.11.004
0033-8389/21/© 2020 Elsevier Inc. All rights reserved.

Anomalies of the visceral mediastinum may be initially detected on chest radiography. Although the identification of small lesions is often difficult, careful examination of the mediastinum on chest radiography may reveal unsuspected abnormalities in otherwise asymptomatic individuals. Mediastinal masses typically present with focal contour abnormalities of the mediastinum or diffuse widening of the mediastinum. Indirect signs with displacement of mediastinal lines and stripes can also be seen. In the case of a hilar or perihilar mass, the hilum overlay sign, which is defined as a visibility of the hilar vasculature through the opacity, suggests that the mass is either within the anterior or posterior compartments. A different sign, the hilum convergence sign, can help to distinguish between pulmonary artery enlargement (manifesting as pulmonary vessels that converge toward the edge of the mass-like opacity) versus a nonvascular hilar mass, such as lung malignancy or lymphadenopathy (in which vessels do not converge toward the edge of the mass-like opacity). If only a frontal radiograph is available, obtaining a lateral radiograph may be helpful in localizing mediastinal anomalies to the proper compartment. After the initial detection of a potential mediastinal lesion, further characterization with cross-sectional imaging is warranted.

Computed tomography (CT) scanning remains the imaging modality of choice to evaluate most mediastinal abnormalities owing to its widespread availability, ability to localize lesions to the correct compartment, and excellent spatial resolution. It can also be used for tissue characterization with detection of macroscopic fat, cystic components, calcification, hemorrhage, and hypervascularity.[3,4] Intravenous (IV) iodinated contrast is usually used, because it allows for an assessment of lesion enhancement and helps in differentiating potential masses from vascular structures.

MR imaging is beneficial for its excellent tissue characterization and lack of ionizing radiation.[5] Thoracic MR imaging provides greater diagnostic precision in the evaluation of indeterminate mediastinal masses on CT scan, such as complex cystic masses or masses containing intralesional fat or hemorrhage.[6,7] It can also be used as a staging study in patients with contrast allergy or renal failure, in whom a contrast-enhanced CT scan may be contraindicated.

Finally, several nuclear medicine studies may be used as additional problem-solving modalities. A PET/CT scan with fluorodeoxyglucose can be used to identify distant metastases in the setting of suspected malignancy.[8] [123]I-Metaiodobenzylguanidine, In-111octreotide scintigraphy, and a PET/CT scan with fluorodeoxyglucose can be used in patients with suspected paragangliomas to further narrow the differential diagnosis. 99mTc pertechnetate scans have a role in the further evaluation of suspected esophageal duplication cysts, where it can accurately localize functioning ectopic gastric mucosa.

## IMAGING FINDINGS AND PATHOLOGY
### Lymphadenopathy

#### Stations
The visceral compartment of the mediastinum includes multiple lymph node stations, including upper and lower paratracheal, subaortic, para-aortic, subcarinal, paraesophageal, and pulmonary ligamental lymph nodes.[9] The enlargement of 1 or more of these lymph nodes may be seen in a wide variety of benign and malignant processes and is the most common cause of a visceral mediastinal mass. A CT scan has greater sensitivity than chest radiography for the detection of lymph node enlargement. A PET/CT scan with fluorodeoxyglucose also plays an important role in evaluation of lymphadenopathy and in directing endobronchial ultrasound-guided biopsies.

#### Appearance and size
On a CT scan, lymph nodes typically appear as oval or round homogeneous masses of soft tissue attenuation in their expected anatomic location. The size criteria for abnormal lymph node enlargement have been discussed in the literature and measurements range from 10 to 15 mm depending on the location.[10,11] The sensitivity and specificity of a CT scan are limited in differentiating malignant and benign lymph node enlargement.[12] However, a CT scan can be used to guide invasive diagnostic procedures and its accessibility makes it a useful modality for monitoring treatment response.

#### Causes of nodal enlargement
Malignant lymphadenopathy can be seen in metastatic disease (from thoracic or extrathoracic primary neoplasms) or lymphoproliferative disorders. Benign enlargement may be seen in the context of pneumonia or pulmonary edema, an inflammatory process like sarcoidosis (**Fig. 1**), or granulomatous infection, or rarer entities like angiofollicular lymph node hyperplasia (Castleman disease, discussed in detail elsewhere in this article). The differential diagnosis can be narrowed by measuring the density of the lymph nodes and evaluating their distribution (**Tables 1** and **2**).

### Lymph Node Attenuation

Hypoattenuating lymph nodes usually represent necrosis and are commonly seen in metastatic disease (**Fig. 2**) or atypical infectious processes

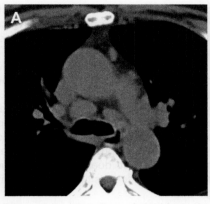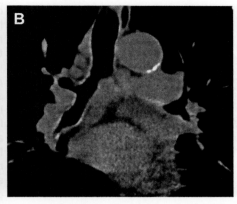

Fig. 1. Sarcoidosis. Axial (*A*) and coronal (*B*) images from an unenhanced CT scan of the chest demonstrates mild enlargement of multiple lymph nodes in the visceral compartment (paratracheal and subcarinal stations).

caused by fungal or mycobacterial agents.[13,14] Much rarer entities include sprue and necrotizing lymphadenitis (Kikuchi–Fujimoto disease).[15]

A hyperattenuating appearance of the lymph nodes may be due to the presence of calcification or mineral dust or due to hypervascularity. The presence of calcifications or other dense inorganic materials can be seen in sarcoidosis, remote granulomatous infection (most commonly tuberculosis and histoplasmosis), treated lymphoproliferative disorders, amyloidosis, and pneumoconioses, such as silicosis and berylliosis.[16] Metastases from thyroid carcinoma and mucinous adenocarcinoma may also calcify.

Hypervascular lymphadenopathy, characterized by brisk enhancement after IV contrast administration, can be seen in metastatic disease, usually from a select group of tumors, including renal cell carcinoma, melanoma, papillary thyroid carcinoma, sarcoma, and neuroendocrine tumors

(Box 1, Table 3). Rarer entities include angiofollicular lymph node hyperplasia (Castleman disease) and Kaposi sarcoma.[17,18] Kikuchi–Fujimoto and Kimura diseases, commonly presenting with cervical lymphadenopathy, can also cause mediastinal lymph node enlargement.[15,19]

## Patterns of Lymph Node Enlargement in Neoplastic and Non-neoplastic Entities

An understanding of lymphatic drainage pathways is helpful in directing attention to relevant stations when interpreting an imaging examination, especially for the staging of cancer. The distribution of lymphadenopathy can also give clues as to the site of the primary tumor in the setting of metastatic disease or suggest alternative diagnoses.

**Table 1**
**Differential diagnosis for multistation lymphadenopathy**

| Category | Possible Causes |
|---|---|
| Neoplastic | Metastases, lymphoproliferative disorders |
| Infectious | Mycobacterial and fungal infection |
| Inflammatory | Sarcoidosis |
| Pneumoconioses | Silicosis, coal worker's pneumoconiosis, berylliosis |
| Reactive | Pulmonary edema, interstitial lung disease |

**Table 2**
**Differential diagnosis for causes of lymphadenopathy based on CT appearance**

| Lymph Node Density | Possible Causes |
|---|---|
| Hypoattenuating | Cystic or necrotic metastases, mycobacterial and fungal infections, lymphoma |
| Hyperattenuating | Sarcoidosis, silicosis and other pneumoconiosis (berylliosis), prior granulomatous infection, amyloidosis, treated lymphoma |
| Hyperenhancing | Hypervascular metastases, Castleman disease, Kaposi sarcoma |

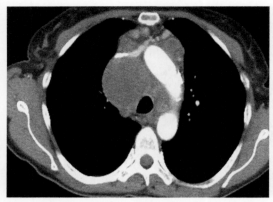

**Fig. 2.** Metastatic lung cancer. A contrast-enhanced axial CT scan of the chest of a patient with lung cancer shows multiple enlarged nodes in the visceral compartment (right paratracheal station) and prevascular mediastinum with central low attenuation and peripheral rim enhancement indicating extensive necrosis. Note the mass effect exerted on adjacent mediastinal structures.

Lung neoplasms usually drain first to the hilar lymph nodes, although direct mediastinal involvement is also possible. Subsequent drainage pathways in the mediastinum depend on the lobe of origin. Right upper lobe tumors drain into the right paratracheal and anterior mediastinal lymph nodes, whereas lesions of the middle and lower lobes drain into the subcarinal lymph nodes before continuing to the right paratracheal lymph nodes. Left upper lobe tumors drain preferentially to the para-aortic and subaortic lymph nodes, whereas those in the left lower lobe favor the subcarinal and subaortic stations.[20]

The upper two-thirds of the esophagus generally drain cranially, whereas the lower one-third drains caudally. Therefore, neoplasia involving the upper two-thirds tend to involve the paratracheal lymph nodes, whereas tumors of the lower one-third preferentially involve the gastrohepatic lymph nodes. The esophageal lymphatics communicate with the thoracic duct; distant nodal metastases are also possible.[21]

Enlargement of the lymph nodes involving multiple mediastinal stations and bilateral hila can be seen in lymphoproliferative disorders. Hodgkin lymphoma in particular involves the mediastinum in up to 85% of cases, especially the superior paratracheal stations and prevascular mediastinum. Non-Hodgkin lymphoma may also involve the mediastinum but does so less frequently and sometimes present as lymphadenopathy in a single station.

Sarcoidosis is a common cause of bilateral hilar lymph node enlargement and should be a leading differential in the absence of known malignancy. Involvement of the paratracheal and subcarinal lymph nodes is also frequent.[22] Pneumoconioses such as silicosis and coal worker's disease can also manifest with a similar distribution, as well as fungal and mycobacterial infections. As outlined elsewhere in this article, measuring the internal density of these lymph nodes may help to narrow the differential diagnosis. Finally, mild diffuse lymph node enlargement can also be seen in reaction to diffuse lung processes, such as pulmonary edema and interstitial lung disease.

### Castleman Disease

Angiofollicular lymph node hyperplasia, also known as Castleman disease (**Fig. 3**), is a rare benign lymphoproliferative disease that frequently presents as a mediastinal mass. Although it can also affect the cervical and abdominal lymph nodes, approximately 70% occur in the chest, and the visceral mediastinum is the most common location.[17,23,24]

Castleman disease has been historically subdivided based on unicentric or multicentric involvement of lymph nodes. However, the modern histopathologic classification recognizes 4 main entities: hyaline vascular Castleman disease, plasma cell Castleman disease, human herpes virus-8–associated Castleman disease, and Castleman disease not otherwise specified. The imaging appearance is typically that of hyperenhancing lymph node enlargement involving 1 or multiple stations. Histologic confirmation is usually necessary for a diagnosis. The differential diagnosis depends on the compartments involved and associated imaging findings. For example, unicentric disease may mimic thymoma, sarcoma, and paraganglioma, whereas multicentric disease resembles lymphoma, metastatic disease, and sarcoidosis, among other diseases.

---

**Box 1**
**Importance of detecting hypervascularity within a visceral mediastinal mass**

Narrows differential diagnosis to a small group of entities.

Entails propensity to bleed and need for careful preprocedure planning, including embolization before any procedure.

Percutaneous biopsy may not be safe; surgical biopsy allowing for better control of hemorrhage may be preferred.

**Table 3**
**Differential diagnosis for hypervascular mediastinal masses**

| Benign | Malignant or Malignant Potential | Metastases |
| --- | --- | --- |
| Castleman's disease | Sarcomas | Renal cell carcinoma |
| Ectopic parathyroid adenoma | Paraganglioma | Thyroid carcinoma |
| Vascular malformations | Carcinoid | Melanoma |
| | Castleman's disease | Pheochromocytoma |
| | | Carcinoid |
| | | Choriocarcinoma |

The hyaline vascular variant comprises 90% of cases and most commonly manifests as unicentric disease, presenting as a solitary hyperenhancing mass in a young adult. The differential diagnosis depends on the affected mediastinal compartment and includes thymoma, lymphoma, sarcoma, and neurogenic tumors. In the absence of IV contrast, complicated foregut duplication cysts may have a similar appearance.

The plasma cell variant most commonly presents as multicentric disease and tends to involve older adults. Lymph node enlargement involving multiple mediastinal compartments and bilateral hila is seen although enhancement following IV contrast administration is reportedly less than that for the hyaline variant. The main differential diagnosis is lymphoma and other causes of multi-station lymphadenopathy, such as sarcoidosis and metastatic disease. Systemic manifestations such as fever, night sweats, and anemia are more common, and the entity has been linked to lymphocytic interstitial pneumonitis.[25]

Human herpes virus-8–associated Castleman disease has a poor prognosis and typically affects immunocompromised patients. It commonly presents as multicentric disease with severe systemic manifestations. The imaging appearance is similar to an aggressive form of plasma cell Castleman disease.

### Trachea
**Bronchogenic cyst** Bronchogenic cysts are congenital foregut malformations typically presenting as well-circumscribed masses with homogeneous internal fluid attenuation and thin or imperceptible wall.[26] Up to 90% are in the visceral mediastinum, usually close to the carina or in the right paratracheal space, although intrapulmonary cysts are also possible.[27] The internal density is usually that of fluid, but variable proteinaceous, mucoid, or hemorrhagic content may increase attenuation, making the distinction between a cyst and a soft tissue mass difficult.[28] After IV contrast administration, the wall may enhance, but there should be no enhancing component within the mass. Because it is easy to misinterpret hyperattenuating cystic lesions as solid on both noncontrast and contrast-enhanced CT scans,

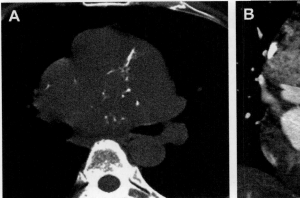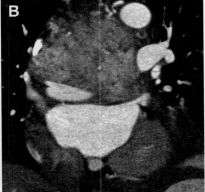

**Fig. 3.** Castleman disease. (*A*) An unenhanced axial CT scan of the chest demonstrates a large solid lobulated visceral mediastinal mass with branching calcifications. (*B*) A contrast-enhanced coronal reformation from a CT scan of the chest shows brisk heterogeneous enhancement with numerous feeding vessels in the periphery of the mass in keeping with the hypervascular nature of the lesion.

the use of MR imaging is critical to make this distinction and prevent unnecessary follow-up and diagnostic interventions. When a mediastinal mass is well-circumscribed, homogeneous in attenuation, and round or oval in configuration, MR imaging should be considered to distinguish between a cystic and a solid lesion.[29] On T2-weighed images, a bronchogenic cyst should have high signal intensity. The T1 signal can be variably high, depending on proteinaceous or hemorrhagic content[30,31] (Fig. 4).

Bronchogenic cysts should not normally communicate with the bronchial tree and the presence of internal gas may signify a superimposed infection.[32] They may cause symptoms such as cough or recurrent pneumonia through compression of adjacent structures such as the airway. Malignant transformation is possible, but very rare.

The differential diagnosis includes other congenital cystic lesions of the mediastinum, such as esophageal duplication cysts, pericardial cysts, and cystic neurogenic lesions. Abscesses, hematomas, and seromas should be considered in the appropriate clinical setting. Lymphatic malformations can be seen typically in pediatric patients. Finally, neoplasia with cystic components should be considered, particularly when enhancing internal components are seen.

**Tracheal tumors and tumor-like entities** Tracheal neoplasms can be seen on CT scans as a focal thickening of the tracheal wall or nodular lesions that extend into the lumen. The differentiation of benign and malignant lesions is often not possible on imaging alone, unless the lesion is large and results in the invasion of adjacent mediastinal structures. CT scans and virtual bronchoscopy can be used to direct endoscopy for biopsy and definitive diagnosis.[33,34]

Primary malignant neoplasms include squamous cell carcinoma, which is strongly associated with smoking and typically occurs in the distal one-third of the trachea, and adenoid cystic carcinoma (Fig. 5), which is not associated with smoking and usually occurs in the distal trachea and proximal bronchi. Mucoepidermoid carcinoma is typically encountered in young adults and presents as a nodule in the main bronchi or, less commonly, in the trachea. Benign lesions include carcinoid, papilloma, hamartoma, and chondroma.[35] Carcinoid tumors typically present as enhancing endobronchial nodules that may calcify. Tracheal papillomatosis occurs after human papilloma virus infection, either from colonization during birth or rarely from dissemination from laryngeal papillomatosis. A CT scan will demonstrate numerous small nodules in the airways and cavitating lung nodules. Finally,

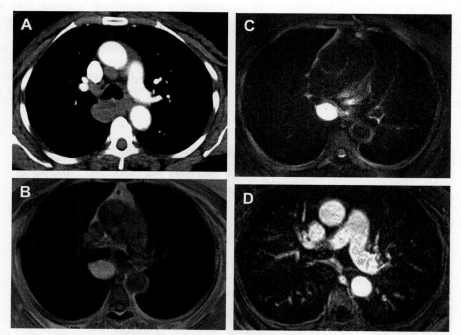

**Fig. 4.** Bronchogenic cyst. (*A*) A contrast-enhanced axial CT scan of the chest shows a round, well-circumscribed, homogeneous, and fluid-attenuating mass in the subcarinal region. Axial T1-weighted (*B*), axial fat-suppressed T2-weighted (*C*), and axial post-contrast T1-weighted (*D*) MR images show a heterogeneous T1 hyperintense and homogeneous T2 hyperintense mass without internal nodularity or septation that does not enhance following the administration of IV gadolinium contrast..

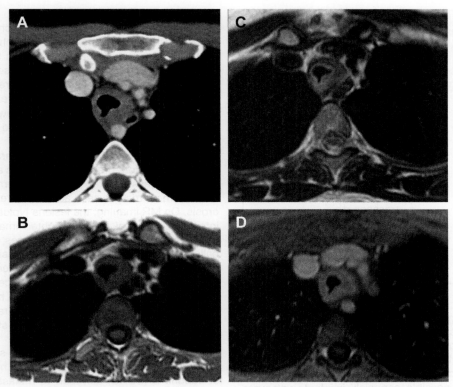

**Fig. 5.** Adenoid cystic carcinoma. (*A*) A contrast-enhanced axial CT image of the chest demonstrates smooth, circumferential and asymmetric thickening of the tracheal wall. Axial T1-weighted (*B*), axial T2-weighted (*C*), and axial post-contrast T1-weighted (*D*) images better demonstrate mural stratification and enhancing tumor.

it is important to consider foreign bodies, especially in pediatric patients.

**Non-neoplastic tracheal disorders** Tracheal strictures can be seen on a CT scan as focal areas of narrowing. They can occur after prolonged endotracheal intubation or from prior infection, surgery, or inhalation injury.[33]

Diffuse tracheal narrowing is seen in tracheomalacia, causing excessive airway collapse during expiration. The diagnosis can be made on a CT scan when there is a 50% or greater decrease in the transverse tracheal diameter during expiration.[36] This entity is to be distinguished from saber-sheath trachea, which is usually seen in chronic obstructive pulmonary disease and is defined as a coronal diameter that is two-thirds of the sagittal diameter.[37]

Tracheobronchomegaly, also known as Mounier–Kuhn syndrome, is a very rare congenital disorder causing diffuse dilatation of the trachea and central bronchi. Affected patients typically present with recurrent infections.[38]

Thickening of the tracheal wall can be seen in a variety of inflammatory conditions (**Table 4**). Relapsing polychondritis causes diffuse smooth thickening that usually spares the posterior wall.[39] In contrast, granulomatosis with polyangiitis can cause circumferential thickening, though airway involvement is uncommon.[40] Tracheopathia osteochondroplastica is a rare disease causing multiple osteocartilaginous nodules in the tracheal submucosa, typically seen as multiple small calcifying nodules sparing the posterior wall. Amyloidosis can have a similar appearance, although the posterior wall is not spared.[35]

*Esophagus*
**Esophageal duplication cyst** Esophageal duplication cysts are rare congenital foregut malformations presenting as well-circumscribed masses near the esophagus or associated with the esophageal wall. They are typically of homogeneous fluid attenuation, although a greater density can be seen with hemorrhage or infection. These complications can be seen particularly when the cyst contains ectopic gastric mucosa, the presence of which makes 99mTc pertechnetate scans helpful in narrowing down the differential diagnosis.[41] As with other congenital cysts, there should be no internal enhancement with IV contrast. On MR imaging, high T2 signal and variable T1 signal

**Table 4**
**Differential diagnosis for tracheal tumors and tumor-like entities**

| Pattern of Involvement | Possible Causes |
|---|---|
| Focal | Malignant: squamous cell carcinoma, adenoid cystic carcinoma, mucoepidermoid carcinoma<br>Benign: carcinoid, hamartoma, foreign body |
| Diffuse | Posterior wall sparing: Relapsing polychondritis, tracheopathia osteochondroplastica<br>Circumferential: Amyloidosis, sarcoidosis, granulomatosis with polyangiitis, papillomatosis |

(depending on the degree of hemorrhagic or proteinaceous content) are typical.

Esophageal duplication cysts may cause symptoms from the compression of adjacent structures, including dysphagia and pain.[32] Airway obstruction is also possible, especially in infants with cysts located superiorly to the carina.[42]

As described elsewhere in this article, the differential diagnosis includes other congenital cystic lesions, abscesses, hematomas, seromas, and cystic neoplasms.

**Other esophageal lesions** The esophagus should be carefully assessed for masses or wall thickening. Circumferential wall thickening can be seen in esophagitis, either from infectious or inflammatory causes, or neoplasia. Asymmetric or nodular thickening raises concern for malignancy, usually squamous cell carcinoma (**Fig. 6**) or adenocarcinoma.[1] Lesions of the distal one-third of the esophagus are more likely to represent adenocarcinoma because of the association with esophageal reflux. The identification of such lesions warrants investigation with endoscopy and possible biopsy for a definitive diagnosis.

Benign lesions, such as papillomas and lipomas, are usually difficult to diagnose on imaging alone because of their small size. Hiatus hernias may mimic a mediastinal mass on chest radiography, although a CT scan is usually diagnostic. Esophageal varices, often seen in the setting of cirrhosis and portal hypertension, manifest as serpiginous vascular structures.

## Neurogenic tumors

Paragangliomas (extra-adrenal pheochromocytomas) arise from chromaffin cells, which are present in the para-aortic ganglia and can therefore present as visceral mediastinal masses, most commonly along the lesser curvature of the aorta.[43] Mediastinal paragangliomas are typically nonsecretory, but those located in the lower mediastinum can be secretory and can lead to catecholamine excess.[44]

Paragangliomas tend to be highly vascular tumors and therefore present on CT scans as briskly enhancing masses (**Fig. 7**). Areas of internal hypoenhancement may be seen and correlate with necrosis. On MR imaging, the lesions typically show intermediate signal on T1-weighted images and hyperintensity on T2-weighted images (the so-called light bulb sign). Foci of hypointensity corresponding with flow voids may also be seen with a resultant salt and pepper appearance.[45] [123]I-metaiodobenzylguanidine can also be helpful in narrowing the differential. Malignant paragangliomas can be seen to invade nearby structures and cause metastasis.[46]

Paragangliomas are associated with succinate dehydrogenase mutations. In particular, mutations of subunit B (SDHB) can lead to metastatic disease in more than 40% of patients.[47] MR imaging is favored to monitor patients with known SDHB mutation owing to the lack of associated ionizing radiation.

## Mesenchymal lesions

**Lesions of adipose tissue** Mediastinal lipomatosis and lipomas are benign entities that can be diagnosed on imaging. Lipomatosis refers to increased fat in the mediastinum without a surrounding capsule, whereas a lipoma is an encapsulated and well-circumscribed fat-containing mass. In both cases, the fat content should be homogeneous and follow subcutaneous fat density on CT scans and signal on MR imaging.[48]

Mediastinal liposarcomas are malignant tumors that can rarely arise in the visceral mediastinum (**Fig. 8**). They tend to appear heterogeneous with internal soft tissue densities on CT scan. MR imaging is particularly useful at demonstrating intralesional fat, appearing hyperintense on T1- and T2-weighted images and hypointense on saturated sequences, with interspersed enhancing soft tissue. A mass effect and invasion of adjacent structures can also be seen.[49,50]

**Other mesenchymal tumors** Hemangiomas are benign vascular neoplasms, whereas vascular malformations represent a wide variety of nonneoplastic vascular lesions. These entities are

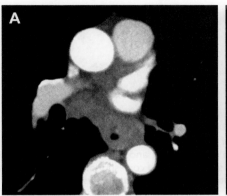
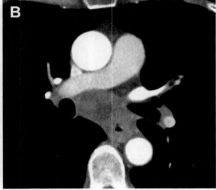

**Fig. 6.** Squamous cell carcinoma of the esophagus. Axial images from a contrast-enhanced chest CT demonstrating asymmetric thickening of the esophageal wall (*A*) and necrotic subcarinal lymphadenopathy (*B*).

very rare in the visceral mediastinum. Hemangiomas present as enhancing masses, whereas vascular malformations have a wide range of appearance depending on the involved vessels and lymphatics. Other rare entities include mediastinal fibromatosis, solitary fibrous tumors, inflammatory myofibroblastic tumor and sarcomas.

### Mediastinitis

Mediastinitis (**Fig. 9**) involving the visceral mediastinum can be seen after traumatic or iatrogenic damage to the esophagus or airway.[51] It may also be seen as a complication of cardiothoracic surgery. The spread of infection from adjacent compartments, particularly from the neck into the superior mediastinum, may also extend into the visceral mediastinum.

Although mediastinitis and abscesses can be suggested by mediastinal widening on chest radiography, CT scanning is the imaging modality of choice and demonstrates diffuse fat stranding. A fluid collection with enhancing walls and gas content is suggestive of an abscess.[51] Air bubbles

may suggest airway or esophageal perforation, and these structures must then be carefully assessed to identify the potential origin of the leak. Using water-soluble oral contrast is useful in localizing an esophageal leak and can be used to direct endoscopy procedures.[52] The differential diagnosis includes postoperative edema or hemorrhage, either from surgery or trauma.

### Other complex cystic lesions

Cystic mediastinal masses include a wide range of congenital, developmental, infectious, inflammatory, and neoplastic processes. Although some cystic masses can be definitively diagnosed on CT scans, others remain indeterminate. Because of its intrinsic superior soft tissue resolution, MR imaging is an important tool in the evaluation of select mediastinal masses that are incompletely characterized on CT scanning. Besides complex bronchopulmonary foregut duplication cysts, cystic lymphangiomas and tumors with cystic degeneration described elsewhere in this article, miscellaneous entities such as postoperative

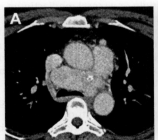
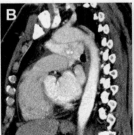
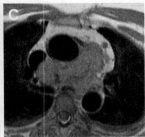

**Fig. 7.** Paraganglioma. A contrast-enhanced axial (*A*) and sagittal (*B*) CT scan of the chest demonstrates an avidly enhancing mass in the aortopulmonary window in close proximity to the inferior aspect of the aortic arch and superior aspect of the pulmonary arteries. The mass contains several calcifications. (*C*) Black blood double inversion recovery (DIR) axial MR image shows the invasive nature of the mass.

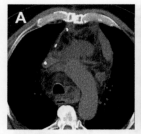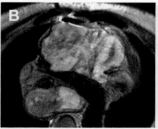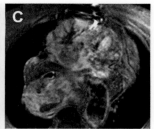

**Fig. 8.** Liposarcoma. (*A*) An unenhanced axial CT scan of the chest shows an infiltrative mass involving multiple compartments, including the visceral mediastinum, with regions of fat and soft tissue attenuation. (*B*) Axial T2-weighted MR image demonstrates internal foci of high signal intensity corresponding to fat. (*C*) Axial postcontrast T1-weighed MR image shows heterogeneous enhancement throughout the lesion.

hematomas and seromas and pancreatic pseudo-cysts can also present as cystic lesions within the visceral compartment. Occasionally, a high riding superior aortic recess of the pericardium may also mimic a cystic lesion or necrotic adenopathy in the right paratracheal region.

### Lesions originating from other mediastinal compartments

Although dividing the mediastinum in compartments is helpful in establishing a differential diagnosis, it is important to keep in mind that lesions may transgress a given compartment. In the setting of a very large mass, identifying its point of origin may prove to be difficult. Thus, lesions originating in either the prevascular or paravertebral mediastinum must be kept in mind when faced with a visceral mediastinal mass. Additionally, lung masses may also invade the visceral mediastinum.

## SUMMARY

Accurate identification and characterization of a mass in the visceral mediastinum usually allows for the development of a focused differential diagnosis. Although lymphadenopathy is the most common process, a select group of other identities can often be diagnosed on imaging by using a variety of modalities. Imaging also plays a key role in guiding invasive diagnostic procedures and monitoring treatment response.

## CLINICS CARE POINTS

**Fig. 9.** Mediastinitis. A contrast-enhanced axial CT scan of the chest demonstrates diffuse infiltration of the mediastinal fat surrounding the trachea and esophagus in this patient with dysphagia and fevers, consistent with the diagnosis of mediastinitis. Endoscopy did not identify esophageal perforation. The patient was treated empirically with antibiotics and the findings resolved on subsequent imaging.

- The middle or visceral mediastinum is located between the thoracic inlet and the diaphragm in the craniocaudal axis and between the anterior aspect of the pericardium and a vertical line situated 1 cm posteriorly to the anterior margin of the vertebral bodies in the anteroposterior axis.

- Chest radiography, CT scans, MR imaging, and nuclear medicine studies can be used to detect, characterize, and diagnose abnormalities in this compartment. Imaging also plays an important role in directing invasive diagnostic procedures and monitoring the treatment response.

- Lymphadenopathy is the most common disease process involving the visceral mediastinum. Common malignant causes include metastases and lymphoproliferative disorders. Benign causes include infection (particularly from mycobacterial and fungal agents), sarcoidosis, and pneumoconioses.

- Foregut malformations such as bronchogenic cysts and esophageal duplication cysts are rare entities that may present as homogeneous cystic masses with no internal enhancement. In many cases, they can be reliably diagnosed on imaging alone. Potential pitfalls include increased attenuation from hemorrhagic or proteinaceous content and wall enhancement, which may prompt further evaluation with MR imaging.

- Paragangliomas, which can be nonsecretory or secretory and lead to catecholamine excess, may occur in the visceral mediastinum and manifest as avidly enhancing masses in close proximity to the great vessels.

- Neoplasms of the trachea and esophagus may be difficult to identify because of their small size and differentiation between malignant and benign entities is often not possible on imaging alone. The main role of imaging is to detect these anomalies, direct endoscopy, and monitor treatment response.

- Mediastinitis, with or without abscess, may occur after esophageal or airway perforation, cardiothoracic surgery, or trauma. A CT scan can be used to investigate for possible complications.

## DISCLOSURE

The authors have nothing to disclose.

## REFERENCES

1. Carter BW, Benveniste MF, Madan R, et al. ITMIG classification of mediastinal compartments and multidisciplinary approach to mediastinal masses. Radiographics 2017;37(2):413–36.
2. Carter BW, Tomiyama N, Bhora FY, et al. A modern definition of mediastinal compartments. J Thorac Oncol 2014;9(9 Suppl 2):S97–101.
3. Reiser M. Multidetector-row CT of the Thorax. Springer-Verlag Berlin Heidelberg: Springer Science & Business Media; 2004.
4. Rydberg J, Buckwalter KA, Caldemeyer KS, et al. Multisection CT: scanning techniques and clinical applications. Radiographics 2000;20(6):1787–806.
5. Broncano J, Alvarado-Benavides AM, Bhalla S, et al. Role of advanced magnetic resonance imaging in the assessment of malignancies of the mediastinum. World J Radiol 2019;11(3):27–45.
6. Ackman JB. MR imaging of mediastinal masses. Magn Reson Imaging Clin N Am 2015;23(2):141–64.
7. Carter BW, Betancourt SL, Benveniste MF. MR imaging of mediastinal masses. Top Magn Reson Imaging 2017;26(4):153–65.
8. Kubota K, Yamada S, Kondo T, et al. PET imaging of primary mediastinal tumours. Br J Cancer 1996;73(7):882–6.
9. El-Sherief AH, Lau CT, Wu CC, et al. International association for the study of lung cancer (IASLC) lymph node map: radiologic review with CT illustration. Radiographics 2014;34(6):1680–91.
10. Staples CA, Müller NL, Miller RR, et al. Mediastinal nodes in bronchogenic carcinoma: comparison between CT and mediastinoscopy. Radiology 1988;167(2):367–72.
11. McLoud TC, Bourgouin PM, Greenberg RW, et al. Bronchogenic carcinoma: analysis of staging in the mediastinum with CT by correlative lymph node mapping and sampling. Radiology 1992;182(2):319–23.
12. Prenzel KL, Mönig SP, Sinning JM, et al. Lymph node size and metastatic infiltration in non-small cell lung cancer. Chest 2003;123(2):463–7.
13. Suwatanapongched T, Gierada DS. CT of thoracic lymph nodes. Part II: diseases and pitfalls. Br J Radiol 2006;79(948):999–1000.
14. Im JG, Song KS, Kang HS, et al. Mediastinal tuberculous lymphadenitis: CT manifestations. Radiology 1987;164(1):115–9.
15. Błasiak P, Jeleń M, Rzechonek A, et al. Histiocytic necrotising lymphadenitis in mediastinum mimicking thymoma or lymphoma - case presentation and literature review of Kikuchi Fujimoto disease. Polish J Pathol 2016;67(1):91–5 [quiz: 96].
16. Gross BH, Schneider HJ, Proto AV. Eggshell calcification of lymph nodes: an update. AJR Am J Roentgenol 1980;135(6):1265–8.
17. McAdams HP, Rosado-de-Christenson M, Fishback NF, et al. Castleman disease of the thorax: radiologic features with clinical and histopathologic correlation. Radiology 1998;209(1):221–8.
18. Herts BR, Megibow AJ, Birnbaum BA, et al. High-attenuation lymphadenopathy in AIDS patients: significance of findings at CT. Radiology 1992;185(3):777–81.
19. Kumar V, Mittal N, Huang Y, et al. A case series of Kimura's disease: a diagnostic challenge. Ther Adv Hematol 2018;9(7):207–11.
20. Sharma A, Fidias P, Hayman LA, et al. Patterns of lymphadenopathy in thoracic malignancies. Radiographics 2004;24(2):419–34.
21. Riquet M, Saab M, Le Pimpec Barthes F, et al. Lymphatic drainage of the esophagus in the adult. Surg Radiol Anat 1993;15(3):209–11.

22. Criado E, Sánchez M, Ramírez J, et al. Pulmonary sarcoidosis: typical and atypical manifestations at high-resolution CT with pathologic correlation. Radiographics 2010;30(6):1567–86.

23. Bonekamp D, Horton KM, Hruban RH, et al. Castleman disease: the great mimic. Radiographics 2011; 31(6):1793–807.

24. Kligerman SJ, Auerbach A, Franks TJ, et al. Castleman disease of the thorax: clinical, radiologic, and pathologic correlation: from the radiologic pathology archives. Radiographics 2016;36(5):1309–32.

25. Johkoh T, Müller NL, Ichikado K, et al. Intrathoracic multicentric Castleman disease: CT findings in 12 patients. Radiology 1998;209(2):477–81.

26. McAdams HP, Kirejczyk WM, Rosado-de-Christenson ML, et al. Bronchogenic cyst: imaging features with clinical and histopathologic correlation. Radiology 2000;217(2):441–6.

27. Zylak CJ, Eyler WR, Spizarny DL, et al. Developmental lung anomalies in the adult: radiologic-pathologic correlation. Radiographics 2002;22 Spec No:S25–43.

28. Mendelson DS, Rose JS, Efremidis SC, et al. Bronchogenic cysts with high CT numbers. AJR Am J Roentgenol 1983;140(3):463–5.

29. Murayama S, Murakami J, Watanabe H, et al. Signal intensity characteristics of mediastinal cystic masses on T1-weighted MRI. J Comput Assist Tomogr 1995;19(2):188–91.

30. Nakata H, Egashira K, Watanabe H, et al. MRI of bronchogenic cysts. J Comput Assist Tomogr 1993;17(2):267–70.

31. Odev K, Arıbaş BK, Nayman A, et al. Imaging of cystic and cyst-like lesions of the mediastinum with pathologic correlation. J Clin Imaging Sci 2012;2:33.

32. Jeung MY, Gasser B, Gangi A, et al. Imaging of cystic masses of the mediastinum. Radiographics 2002;22 Spec No:S79–93.

33. Miller WT Jr. Obstructive diseases of the trachea. Semin Roentgenol 2001;36(1):21–40.

34. Finkelstein SE, Schrump DS, Nguyen DM, et al. Comparative evaluation of super high-resolution CT scan and virtual bronchoscopy for the detection of tracheobronchial malignancies. Chest 2003;124(5): 1834–40.

35. Shepard JO, Flores EJ, Abbott GF. Imaging of the trachea. Ann Cardiothorac Surg 2018;7(2):197–209.

36. Baroni RH, Feller-Kopman D, Nishino M, et al. Tracheobronchomalacia: comparison between end-expiratory and dynamic expiratory CT for evaluation of central airway collapse. Radiology 2005;235(2): 635–41.

37. Ciccarese F, Poerio A, Stagni S, et al. Saber-sheath trachea as a marker of severe airflow obstruction in chronic obstructive pulmonary disease. Radiol Med 2014;119(2):90–6.

38. Shin MS, Jackson RM, Ho KJ. Tracheobronchomegaly (Mounier-Kuhn syndrome): CT diagnosis. AJR Am J Roentgenol 1988;150(4):777–9.

39. Lee KS, Ernst A, Trentham DE, et al. Relapsing polychondritis: prevalence of expiratory CT airway abnormalities. Radiology 2006;240(2):565–73.

40. Stein MG, Gamsu G, Webb WR, et al. Computed tomography of diffuse tracheal stenosis in Wegener granulomatosis. J Comput Assist Tomogr 1986; 10(5):868–70.

41. Ferguson CC, Young LN, Sutherland JB, et al. Intrathoracic gastrogenic cyst–preoperative diagnosis by technetium pertechnetate scan. J Pediatr Surg 1973;8(5):827–8.

42. Macpherson RI. Gastrointestinal tract duplications: clinical, pathologic, etiologic, and radiologic considerations. Radiographics 1993;13(5):1063–80.

43. Buchanan SN, Radecki KM, Chambers LW. Mediastinal paraganglioma. Ann Thorac Surg 2017;103(5): e413–4.

44. Else T, Greenberg S, Fishbein L. Hereditary paraganglioma-pheochromocytoma syndromes. In: Adam MP, Ardinger HH, Pagon RA, et al, editors. GeneReviews(®). Seattle (WA): University of Washington, Seattle; 1993. p. 6. Copyright © 1993-2020, University of Washington, Seattle. GeneReviews is a registered trademark of the University of Washington, Seattle. All rights reserved.

45. Olsen WL, Dillon WP, Kelly WM, et al. MR imaging of paragangliomas. AJR Am J Roentgenol 1987; 148(1):201–4.

46. Wald O, Shapira OM, Murar A, et al. Paraganglioma of the mediastinum: challenges in diagnosis and surgical management. J Cardiothorac Surg 2010;5: 19.

47. Lenders JW, Duh QY, Eisenhofer G, et al. Pheochromocytoma and paraganglioma: an endocrine society clinical practice guideline. J Clin Endocrinol Metab 2014;99(6):1915–42.

48. Boiselle PM, Rosado-de-Christenson ML. Fat attenuation lesions of the mediastinum. J Comput Assist Tomogr 2001;25(6):881–9.

49. Miura K, Hamanaka K, Matsuoka S. Primary mediastinal dedifferentiated liposarcoma: five case reports and a review. Thorac Cancer 2018;9(12):1733–40.

50. Stark P, Eber CD, Jacobson F. Primary intrathoracic malignant mesenchymal tumors: pictorial essay. J Thorac Imaging 1994;9(3):148–55.

51. Carrol CL, Jeffrey RB Jr, Federle MP, et al. CT evaluation of mediastinal infections. J Comput Assist Tomogr 1987;11(3):449–54.

52. Madan R, Laur O, Crudup B, et al. Imaging of iatrogenic oesophageal injuries using optimized CT oesophageal leak protocol: pearls and pitfalls. Br J Radiol 2018;91(1083):20170629.

# Esophageal Neoplasms
## Radiologic-Pathologic Correlation

John P. Lichtenberger III, MD[a],*, Merissa N. Zeman, MD[b],
Adam R. Dulberger, MD, Capt, USAF, MC[c], Sadiq Alqutub, MD[d], Brett W. Carter, MD[e],
Maria A. Manning, MD[f,g]

## KEYWORDS

- Esophageal neoplasms • Esophagus • Radiologic-pathologic correlation • Computed tomography
- Magnetic resonance imaging • FDG PET/CT

## KEY POINTS

- The radiologic-pathologic correlation of esophageal neoplasms is an important skill for clinical imagers, informing both diagnosis and anticipated clinical management.
- The epidemiology and management of esophageal carcinomas are changing, and clinical imagers will have increased specificity and clinical relevancy if they can put these tumors into an appropriate clinical context.
- Rare malignancies and benign esophageal neoplasms have distinct imaging appearances because of their underlying histology.

## INTRODUCTION

Esophageal cancer is the seventh most common cancer worldwide, with more than 572,000 cases, resulting in more than 508,000 deaths in 2018.[1] In the United States in 2020, the American Cancer Society estimates there will be more than 18,400 new cases of esophageal cancer diagnosed, resulting in more than 16,000 deaths.[2] Although esophageal squamous cell carcinoma (ESCC) accounts for approximately 90% of cases worldwide, largely attributable to cigarette smoking and alcohol consumption, there has been a shift toward esophageal adenocarcinomas (EACs), especially in North America and Europe.[3] In the United States, the prevalence of EAC has now surpassed that of ESCC, as the prevalence of gastroesophageal reflux disease (GERD) and prevalence of obesity have increased.[4–6]

At autopsy, benign tumors represent only 20% of esophageal neoplasms.[7] Most are small lesions that cause no symptoms; however, dysphagia, bleeding, or other symptoms can occur, in which case endoscopic or surgical removal may be necessary. Of these, leiomyomas occur most frequently, accounting for more than 50% of all benign neoplasms, and occur nearly twice as often in men.[8,9] Tumor-like conditions, such as fibrovascular polyps, also occur in the esophagus and have a distinct clinical presentation and imaging appearance.

This article examines the imaging appearances of esophageal neoplasms, with an emphasis on the pathologic basis of those manifestations. Although accurate diagnosis of esophageal neoplasms typically begins with imaging, the pathologic findings play a key role in determining treatment and

[a] The George Washington University Medical Faculty Associates, 900 23rd Street Northwest, Suite G 2092, Washington, DC 20037, USA; [b] Department of Radiology, The George Washington University Hospital, 900 23rd Street Northwest, Suite G 2092, Washington, DC 20037, USA; [c] Department of Radiology, David Grant Medical Center, Travis Air Force Base, 101 Bodin Cir, Fairfield, CA 94533, USA; [d] Department of Pathology, The George Washington University Hospital, 900 23rd Street Northwest, Suite G 2092, Washington, DC 20037, USA; [e] Department of Thoracic Imaging, MD Anderson Cancer Center, 1515 Holcombe Boulevard, Unit 1478, Houston, TX 77030, USA; [f] American Institute for Radiologic Pathology, American College of Radiology, 1100 Wayne Avenue, Suite 1020, Silver Spring, MD 20910, USA; [g] MedStar Georgetown University Hospital, Washington, DC, USA
* Corresponding author.
E-mail address: jlichtenberger@mfa.gwu.edu

Radiol Clin N Am 59 (2021) 205–217
https://doi.org/10.1016/j.rcl.2020.11.002
0033-8389/21/© 2020 Elsevier Inc. All rights reserved.

prognosis, and imagers should be equipped to discuss this radiologic-pathologic relationship as part of the care team.

## ESOPHAGEAL SQUAMOUS CELL CARCINOMA
### Clinical Features

ESCC is a malignant epithelial tumor of the esophagus with squamous cell differentiation. The etiology of ESCC is multifactorial and has been shown to be strongly population-dependent.[6] In the United States, the 2 most significant risk factors are tobacco use and excessive alcohol consumption, which together have a synergistic effect. Certain medical conditions, including Fanconi anemia, lye strictures, Plummer-Vinson syndrome, Zenker diverticulum, tylosis, achalasia, and prior therapeutic radiation to the chest, also place patients at higher risk for ESCC.[10]

ESCC has a male predominance and is 5 times more common among African Americans than whites.[10] The median age of presentation is within the seventh decade of life. Patients tend to be asymptomatic early in the disease, but, by the time of presentation, 80% to 90% of patients endorse progressive dysphagia (Hofstetter, 2019).[10] Weight loss results from decreased oral intake and is associated with worse clinical outcomes.[10] Other symptoms include odynophagia, emesis, cough, chest pain, and anemia.

Local tumor extension can manifest as hoarseness secondary to recurrent laryngeal nerve injury or, occasionally, as an esophagorespiratory fistula. Rarely, ESCC patients may demonstrate hypercalcemia secondary to tumoral production of parathyroid hormone–related protein. Distant metastases may be seen in up to 20% to 30% of patients at presentation.[11] The most common locations of distant metastases include the lungs, liver, bones, and brain. Synchronous or metachronous head/neck SCCs are present in 3% to 10% of patients, which are thought to be related to smoking.[12]

### Pathologic Reatures

ESCC develops through a stepwise progression from histologically normal squamous mucosa to squamous cell dysplasia and finally to invasive squamous cell carcinoma. Squamous cell dysplasia (or intraepithelial neoplasia) is considered a histologic precursor and is characterized by cellular atypia, abnormal differentiation, and disorganized architecture.[12,13] Not only is intraepithelial neoplasia found adjacent to invasive ESCC in a majority of cases, but also its presence at biopsy places a patient at significantly increased risk for the future development of ESCC.

With neoplastic cell invasion through the basement membrane, a lesion is considered invasive ESCC. Defining tumor depth of invasion on a microscopic level is an important prognostic factor. As tumor invasion becomes progressively deeper, there is a concomitant increase in frequency of lymph node metastases.[12] The frequency of lymph node metastases nearly doubles as a tumor invades into each progressively deeper one-third of the submucosal layer.[14]

### Imaging Features

Multimodality imaging plays a crucial role in the clinical staging of ESCC and treatment planning (Figs. 1 and 2). Clinical staging is defined by the American Joint Committee on Cancer staging system using TNM subclassifications, which is currently in its eighth edition, for esophageal and esophagogastric carcinomas.[15] Tumor location no longer is considered a factor in determining clinical staging but should be noted, because it determines the expected location of potential regional lymph node metastases and can have an impact on surgical approach. With imaging and endoscopy, the tumor's epicenter rather than its upper edge is described. A majority of ESCCs are located within the mid-esophagus followed by the lower esophagus.

Traditionally, barium esophagography was considered part of the work-up for esophageal carcinomas. This examination no longer is considered routine but occasionally may be performed prior to endoscopies, acting as a road map. On double-contrast esophagrams, superficial tumors appear as small protruded lesions, manifesting as plaque-like lesions with or without central ulcers, sessile polyps, and/or focal irregularities of the esophageal wall.[16] The more commonly seen advanced tumors are infiltrating, manifesting as irregular luminal narrowing with nodularity and/or ulceration and abrupt shouldering margins.[16,17] Morphology on barium studies typically matches those on endoscopy and pathology,[14] and, although not specific, occasionally can suggest depth of invasion and risk of lymph node metastases.[18]

Computed tomography (CT) is an important modality in the work-up of esophageal cancers. Primary tumors are detected on CT through evaluation of esophageal wall thickness, which is considered abnormal if greater than 5 mm.[15] ESCC typically manifests as esophageal wall thickening or a mass that causes luminal obstruction if advanced. Earlier tumors may be difficult to detect but occasionally can present as asymmetric thickening of the esophageal wall. Beyond displaying

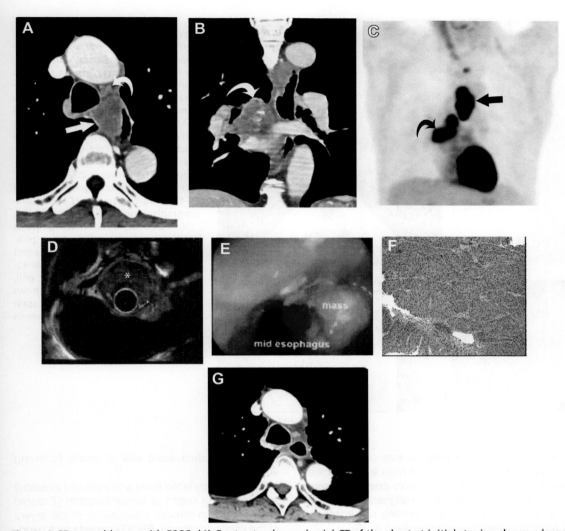

**Fig. 1.** A 67-year-old man with ESCC. (*A*) Contrast-enhanced axial CT of the chest at initial staging shows a large hypoattenuating mass in the right anterolateral esophageal wall in the mid-esophagus (*straight arrow*) and small left paratracheal lymph node adjacent to the mass (*curved arrow*). (*B*) Coronal reformatted contrast-enhanced CT of the chest shows subcarinal lymphadenopathy (*curved arrow*) compatible with locoregional spread. (*C*) Maximum intensity projection (MIP) image from the initial FDG PET/CT shows a hypermetabolic mid-esophageal mass with a SUVmax of 9.0 (*straight arrow*) and moderately hypermetabolic locoregional disease (*curved arrow*). (*D*) EUS shows a large hypoechoic mass in the mid-esophagus that extends through the muscularis propria without invasion into adjacent organs (*asterisk*), compatible with T3 staging. (*E*) EGD demonstrates a near-circumferential mid-esophageal mass, which appears polypoid and contains ulcerated, friable surfaces. (*F*) Photomicrograph (original magnification, ×4; hematoxylin-eosin stain) of a section from the patient's biopsy shows an infiltrative tumor composed of cohesive nests of tumor cells consistent with invasive keratinizing squamous cell carcinoma arising in a background of high-grade squamous dysplasia. (*G*) Contrast-enhanced axial CT of the chest following neoadjuvant chemoradiation illustrates a good response to treatment with near resolution of the mid-esophageal mass and interval decrease in lymphadenopathy.

the primary tumor, CT is unable to illuminate the depth of tumor invasion, particularly in early cancers, significantly limiting its usefulness in T staging.[11] Despite this limitation, CT does have some utility in the assessment of T4 lesions. In general, local invasion is suggested with a loss of fat planes between the tumor and adjacent structures in the mediastinum. For example, if the tumor and aorta have an interface greater than 90°, this can suggest aortic invasion.[19] CT has a moderate sensitivity for detection of locoregional disease and even higher for distant metastases.[10,11] CT evaluation of nodal

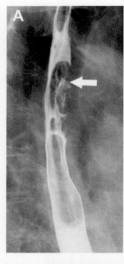
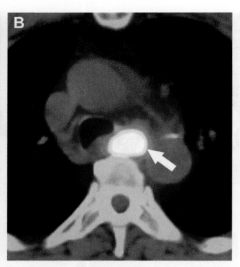
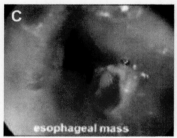
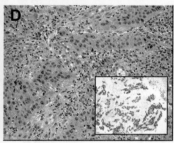

**Fig. 2.** A 57-year-old man with a history of HIV (undetectable viral load) and ESCC. (*A*) Right anterior oblique image from an esophagram shows an infiltrating mass (*arrow*) that has acute, shouldering margins with ulceration and moderate lumen compression. (*B*) Fused axial FDG PET/CT image shows hypermetabolic (SUVmax of 24.9) circumferential thickening of the mid-esophagus (*arrow*). (*C*) Esophagogastroduodenoscopy (EGD) shows a 2.5-cm friable, oozing polypoid mass with ulceration in the mid-esophagus. (*D*) Photomicrograph (original magnification, ×10; hematoxylin-eosin stain) shows markedly atypical cells with amphophilic cytoplasm and no apparent keratin formation, high nuclear-to-cytoplasmic ratio, prominent nucleoli, and anisonucleosis. Inset image shows a positive immunohistochemical stain for p40 supporting squamous differentiation.

disease is based primarily on size criteria, which characterizes a lymph node as pathologic if it measures greater than 1 cm in short-axis in the presence of known esophageal malignancy.[20] This is, however, neither specific or sensitive and is less accurate than endoscopic ultrasound (EUS).

Fluorodeoxyglucose (FDG) PET/CT can delineate the location of the primary tumor, because most ESCCs are FDG-avid. Similar to CT, however, this imaging modality has little role in T staging, because it is unable to differentiate among the different layers of the esophageal wall. It can less commonly delineate locoregional disease[21] but is inferior to EUS. FDG PET/CT's true importance lies in its ability to detect distant metastases and recurrence. It has been shown to be far superior in the detection of distant metastases compared with CT and EUS.[22] Additionally, FDG PET/CT is critical in evaluating treatment response following neoadjuvant chemoradiation, which has been shown to provide prognostic information regarding survival.[23,24] For example, patients whose FDG PET/CT scans demonstrated maximum standardized uptake values that decreased by greater than 50% compared with their pretreatment scans had a longer overall survival and decreased risk of death following surgery.[25]

EUS currently is the most accurate tool available in determining depth of tumor invasion (T stage) because it can directly visualize all of the layers of the esophageal wall. ESCC presents as a hypoechoic mass that, depending on its depth of invasion, obscures 1 or more of the 5 alternating echogenic and hypoechoic lines that represent the normal layers of the esophageal wall. EUS also is the most accurate means for determining N staging, with a reported accuracy rate of 72% to 80% (compared with the 46%–58% accuracy of CT).[10,11] In contrast, EUS has limited value in the assessment of distant metastases and generally is not recommended for treatment response assessment.[25]

## Management

Because a majority of patients present in advanced stages of the disease, the prognosis for ESCC is poor, with a 5-year survival rate of less than 17%.[26] A multidisciplinary approach is considered the mainstay of treatment of ESCC. Esophagectomy alone is recommended for T1-

T2 cancers or patients who cannot tolerate combined modality therapy. Endoscopic techniques, including endoscopic mucosal resection and ablation therapy, can be considered as esophageal-preserving alternatives to surgery in patients with T1a lesions.[24] Patients with T1b lesions generally are not considered candidates for these approaches due to their increased risk of lymph node involvement. That said, more recently, an increasing number of select patients with superficial submucosal invasion T1b lesions with additional favorable features are being treated with endoscopic mucosal resection with good outcomes.[24]

For locally advanced cancers, multimodality therapy is the standard of care and consists of neoadjuvant chemoradiation followed by restaging and consideration for esophagectomy.[25] Adjuvant chemoradiation may benefit some patients with ESCC, particularly if a patient has not previously received neoadjuvant chemoradiation.[10]

Definitive chemoradiation or, less preferably, radiation therapy without subsequent surgery is a possibility for patients who either opt out of or are not candidates for surgery; this approach has been used increasingly to treat ESCC in the cervical and proximal esophagus.[10] Compared with patients who subsequently underwent esophagectomy, those who solely receive definitive chemoradiation have worse locoregional control, but overall survival does not appear to be significantly different between these groups.[25] A palliative approach generally is pursued for patients with T4b tumors or distant metastases, which can include palliative chemoradiation, surgical debulking, and/or esophageal stenting for better symptom control.[24]

## ESOPHAGEAL ADENOCARCINOMA
### Clinical Features

EAC is a malignant epithelial tumor of the esophagus with glandular or mucinous differentiation that typically arises within Barrett esophagus in the lower one-third of the esophagus. It is strongly tied to chronic GERD and the development of Barrett esophagus. The latter is diagnosed in 1% to 2% of the general population and its annual incidence of malignant transformation to EAC is reported to be 0.2% to 0.5% per year.[10,26] Other risk factors in the development of EAC include tobacco smoking and obesity.

Similar to ESCC, EAC demonstrates a slight male predominance and a mean age at presentation within the seventh decade of life. Unlike ESCC, EAC is more common among whites.[6] The clinical presentation generally mirrors that for ESCC. It is, however, more common for patients with EAC to endorse chronic reflux symptoms.[6] Furthermore, patients with EAC are more likely to demonstrate intra-abdominal metastases in contrast to ESCC, which more commonly metastasizes to intrathoracic or cervical sites.[26] The prognosis for EAC is variable but generally tends to be poor, albeit slightly more favorable than that for ESCC.[27]

### Pathologic Features

Grossly, EACs can be described using the same classification system as ESCCs. EAC lesions tend to be infiltrating, polypoid, or ulcerative. If EAC has developed in a background of Barrett esophagus, this can be visualized on endoscopy as reddish mucosa in the distal esophagus compared with the pale grayish color of the normal esophageal squamous cell epithelium.[28,29]

EAC develops through a multistep pathway characterized by a Barrett metaplasia–dysplasia–adenocarcinoma sequence.[29] Less commonly, it develops within heterotopic gastric mucosa or from esophageal mucosal/submucosal glands.[12] Although other types of columnar metaplasia are possible, it is the presence of intestinal metaplasia with goblet cells that specifically defines Barrett esophagus in the United States.[28]

Similar to ESCC, invasive EAC is defined as the invasion of neoplastic cells through the basement membrane. Microscopically, invasive EAC is characterized by mucinous or gland differentiation.[29] The percentage of glandular formation in the carcinoma forms the basis for EAC grading.[28]

### Imaging Features

Similar to ESCC, multimodality imaging is central to the work-up for EAC (Fig. 3). EACs appear similar to ESCCs on each of the imaging modalities. One feature that can suggest one lesion over the other is its location. EAC tends to occur mainly in the distal esophagus and, unlike ESCC, it has a strong predilection for invading the gastric cardia and/or fundus.[7] Another difference is that EACs are more likely to have adjacent strictures secondary to the presence of chronic GERD, a finding that commonly is appreciated on barium esophagrams.[17] Patients with EACs also are more likely to have intra-abdominal metastases, as discussed previously, which tend to be well visualized on FDG PET/CT and CT. Finally, EACs generally are less FDG-avid than ESCCs and tend to be more heterogeneous in their avidity. As was reported for gastric adenocarcinomas, EACs that are poorly differentiated or demonstrate diffuse-type, signet cell, or mucinous patterns

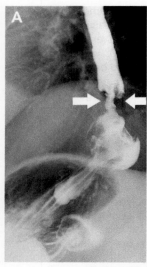
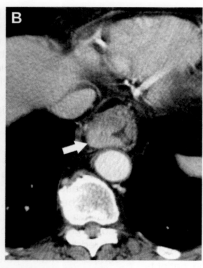

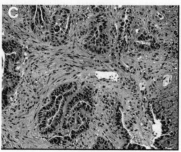

**Fig. 3.** A 78-year-old man with a history of GERD and EAC. (*A*) Oblique image from an esophagram shows an irregular infiltrating mass in the distal esophagus with circumferential stenosis of the lumen and shouldering margins (*arrows*). (*B*) Contrast-enhanced axial CT of the chest at initial staging demonstrates a hypoattenuating mass in the right anterolateral wall of the distal esophagus (*arrow*). (*C*) Photomicrograph (original magnification, ×10; hematoxylin-eosin stain) shows atypical cells lining irregular and incomplete glandular structures, single infiltrating cells, and desmoplastic stromal reaction.

tend to be on average less FDG-avid (Stahl and colleagues, 2008).[30] In general, however, imaging cannot reliably differentiate EAC from ESCC.

## Management

EAC is managed similarly to ESCC with minor differences. For example, because EAC tends to be less radiosensitive compared with ESCC, there is less of a benefit of combined neoadjuvant chemoradiation compared with neoadjuvant chemotherapy alone.[24] Thus, the latter may be considered in patients with EAC. Furthermore, trastuzumab, a humanized monoclonal antibody that targets the human epidermal growth factor receptor family member ERBB2 (HER2), is approved for the treatment of patients with advanced or metastatic HER2-positive EAC. Trastuzumab plus chemotherapy has been shown to improve overall survival in these patients.[31]

## LEIOMYOMAS

Leiomyomas are the most common benign tumors of the esophagus, although they occur approximately 50 times less frequently than esophageal

carcinoma.[32] In contrast to carcinoma, most patients with leiomyomas are asymptomatic, especially patients with tumors less than 5 cm in size.[32] Tumors commonly are detected incidentally on imaging or endoscopy performed for other reasons.

## Pathologic Features

Leiomyomas are neoplasms of mature smooth muscle cells and appear grossly as firm white smoothly marginated masses, with a whorled appearance on cut surface. Tumors almost always are intramural in location, arising from the muscularis mucosae or muscularis propria layers.[32] Microscopically, tumors are composed of bundles of well-differentiated spindled smooth muscle cells.[33] Cells contain abundant eosinophilic neoplasm and are arranged in an interlacing or palisading pattern.[32] Cells have a bland appearance, without mitotic activity or nuclear pleomorphism.[8] On immunohistochemical analysis, lesional cells typically are positive for SMA and desmin, but, unlike gastrointestinal stromal tumors (GISTs), lack affinity for KIT (CD117), CD34, and DOG1.

## Imaging Features

On imaging, esophageal leiomyomas most commonly are an intramural, submucosal mass in the mid to lower esophagus, the portions of the esophagus lined by smooth muscle, and which may distort the azygoesophageal edge (Fig. 4). Barium swallow characteristically demonstrates a smooth-surfaced, crescent-shaped filling defect, which forms obtuse angles with the esophageal wall.[16] These masses may be isoattenuating or hypoattenuating to muscle on unenhanced CT, and they commonly are slightly hyperintense on T2-weighted MR imaging.[8] Homogeneous enhancement, without necrosis, is seen most frequently.[34] Leiomyomas may demonstrate coarse calcification, a feature that helps differentiate them from other benign and malignant esophageal tumors, in which calcification is uncommon.[35,36] FDG PET/CT usually is negative in patients with leiomyomas, attributable to the lack of mitotic activity.[8]

## Management

No cases of sarcomatous degeneration of leiomyoma to leiomyosarcoma have been reported to date.[7] Therefore, surgical removal of small leiomyomas in asymptomatic patients is not performed commonly. Symptomatic lesions, however, may necessitate surgical resection. Although complete resection of a small leiomyosarcoma often can be accomplished through local excision, larger tumors may require a total or partial esophagectomy.[37]

## SARCOMAS

Although sarcomas are uncommon in the esophagus, leiomyosarcoma is the most common type.[8] These tumors are characterized by slow growth and late metastases and are thought to arise de novo rather than from preexisting leiomyomas.[38] Liposarcomas rarely are reported in the esophagus.[39]

## Pathologic Features

On gross examination, leiomyosarcomas arise in the wall of the esophagus and appear as polypoid or lobulated intraluminal tumors, which may feature ulceration.[40] Microscopically, these are cellular tumors, with long intersecting fascicles of spindle cells. Tumor cells contain ample eosinophilic cytoplasm and pleomorphic enlarged nuclei. Increased mitotic activity is common in gastrointestinal leiomyosarcomas, and necrosis may be present.[40]

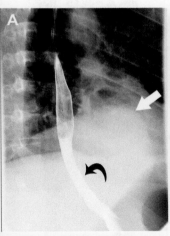
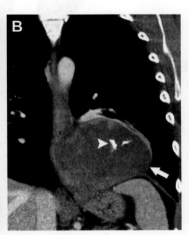
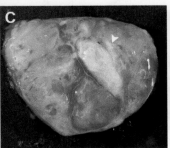
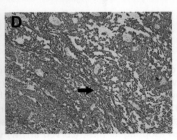

Fig. 4. A 42-year-old man with leiomyoma of the esophagus. (A) Coned-down image from an esophagram shows the contour of a mass (straight arrow) at the left aspect of the esophagus with smooth mass effect on the left aspect of the esophagus (curved arrow). (B) Coronal reformatted contrast-enhanced CT of the chest shows a homogeneous hypoattenuating mass (arrow) contiguous with the esophagus containing internal focus of calcification (arrowhead). (C) Sectioned gross specimen shows a gelatinous tan-red cut surface with partially calcified (arrowhead) necrosis. (D) Photomicrograph (original magnification, ×40; desmin immunohistochemical stain) shows spindle cells (arrow) uniformly positive.

Adipose tissue and fibrous septa are characteristic of liposarcoma of the esophagus, and some liposarcomas may be grossly pedunculated and mimic a fibrovascular polyp histologically, differentiated by irregular spindle cells and MDM2 amplification in liposarcomas.[39]

## Imaging Features

On CT, these malignant tumors are heterogeneous and feature central areas of necrosis. Large exophytic components may cause mass effect on the trachea or other nearby structures. Ulceration may allow extraluminal gas or contrast material to track into the tumor.[41] On MR imaging, these lesions typically are isointense with skeletal muscle on T1-weighted images and hyperintense on T2-weighted images. A central signal void may be present, as the result of extraluminal gas within the tumor.[41] Fat attenuation on CT or chemical fat signal on MR imaging may suggest liposarcoma (Fig. 5).

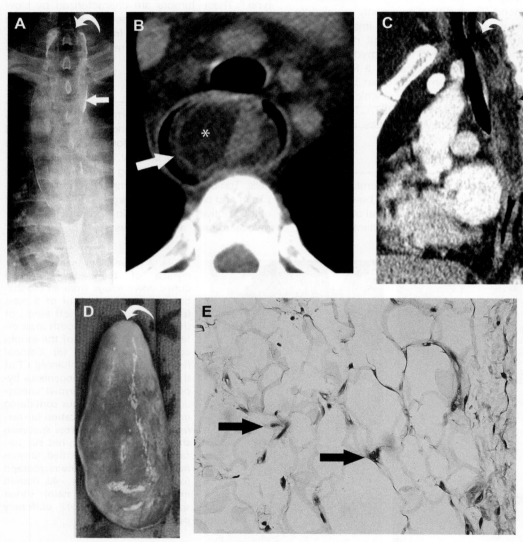

**Fig. 5.** A 39-year-old man with liposarcoma of the esophagus. (*A*) Coned-down image from an esophagram shows a mass (*straight arrow*) filling the esophagus with stalk-like attachment at the cervical esophagus (*curved arrow*). (*B*) Contrast-enhanced axial CT of the chest shows the esophageal mass (*arrow*) with extensive fat attenuation component (*asterisk*) and soft tissue nodularity. (*C*) Sagittal reformatted contrast-enhanced CT of the chest image shows a polypoid esophageal mass (*arrows*) with stalk-like attachment at the upper esophagus (*curved arrow*). (*D*) Gross specimen shows an elongated, encapsulated esophageal mass (*curved arrow*) with macroscopic fat most notably at the superior aspect near its attachment to the cervical esophagus. (*E*) Photomicrograph (hematoxylin-eosin, original magnification ×40) shows mild atypia of adipocytes with enlarged, hyperchromic nuclei (*arrows*).

## Management

Five-year survival rates of approximately 30% to 40% are reported in patients with surgically resected leiomyosarcoma, and survival is influenced strongly by tumor differentiation and size.[42] Tumors eventually may spread by direct extension to the pleura, pericardium, diaphragms, and stomach or metastasize hematogenously to the liver, lungs, and bones.[7]

## GASTROINTESTINAL STROMAL TUMORS

Until recently, almost all mesenchymal neoplasms arising from the esophagus were thought to be benign esophageal leiomyomas.[7] It is now known that another stromal tumor, GISTs, also may occur in the esophagus. Differentiation is important, because of the known malignant potential of GISTs, which warrants consideration for surgical resection or treatment with tyrosine kinase inhibitors, such as imatinib.[43] Although GISTs can occur anywhere in the gastrointestinal tract, most commonly in the stomach, approximately 1% arise in the esophagus.[44] When occurring in the esophagus, these tumors most commonly involve the lower third.

## Pathologic Features

Similar to GISTs elsewhere, small tumors often are intramural and arise in the muscularis propria, whereas larger tumors may exhibit exophytic growth and areas of necrosis.[36] Immunohistochemical analysis often is required to differentiate esophageal leiomyomas from GISTs, because both may demonstrate spindle cells and calcification on histology. Positivity for KIT (CD117), DOG1, and CD34 are more consistent with GIST.[8]

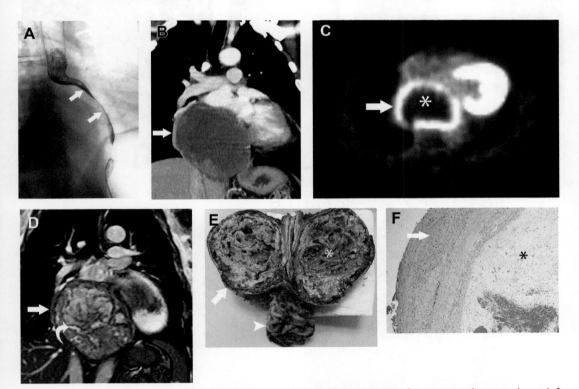

Fig. 6. A 72-year-old man with GIST of the esophagus. (A) Coned-down image from an esophagram shows leftward deviation (*arrows*) of the esophagus without mucosal ulceration, characteristic of mesenchymal tumors of the esophagus. (B) Coronal reformatted contrast-enhanced CT of the chest shows the mass (*arrow*) with peripheral enhancement and central hypoattenuation indicating necrosis. (C) Axial FDG PET shows the mass (*arrow*) with peripheral uptake and no central uptake (*asterisk*), indicating central necrosis. (D) Coronal T2-weighted MR image shows the mass (*straight arrow*) with central heterogeneous and hyperintense regions (*curved arrow*) indicating necrosis or hemorrhage products. (E) Esophagogastrectomy specimen transected in the coronal plane show the mass (*arrow*) arising from the esophagus and extending to the origin of the stomach (*arrowhead*). Note the extensive intratumoral hemorrhage and necrosis (*asterisk*). (F) Photomicrograph (original magnification, ×4; hematoxylin-eosin stain) shows peripheral epithelioid and spindle cells (*arrow*) characteristic of GIST with extensive necrosis and hemorrhage (*asterisk*) centrally.

## Imaging Features

Esophageal GISTs have a similar clinical, endo-scopic, and imaging appearance to leiomyomas. Features that favor GIST over leiomyoma include more distal location, larger size, more heteroge-neous appearance, greater enhancement on contrast-enhanced CT, and marked avidity on FDG PET/CT (Fig. 6).[43] In some cases, EUS-guided fine-needle aspiration for immunohistochemical staining may be required for differentiation. Imaging appearance also may be similar to sarcomas, with areas of necrosis and calcification resulting in het-erogeneous attenuation.[35]

## FIBROVASCULAR POLYPS

Fibrovascular polyps include a variety of lesions, which are differentiated by the predominant

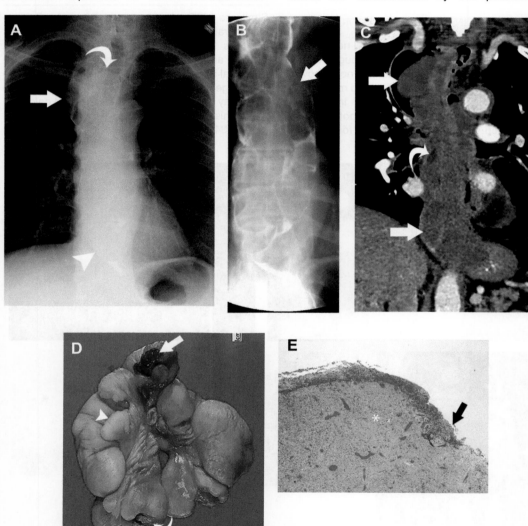

Fig. 7. A 59-year-old man with a fibrovascular polyp of the esophagus. (A) Frontal chest radiograph shows opac-ity at the right paratracheal stripe (straight arrow), an abnormal air-soft tissue interface at the upper medias-tinum (curved arrow), and an abnormal edge near the gastroesophageal junction (arrowhead), indicating esophageal pathology. (B) Coned-down image from an esophagram shows a polypoid mass (arrow) filling the esophagus and outlined in barium without mucosal abnormality. (C) Coronal reformatted contrast-enhanced CT of the chest shows the polypoid mass (straight arrows) filling and distending the esophagus with a small focus of fat attenuation (curved arrow). (D) Gross specimen shows the cut stalk (straight arrow), regions of ulceration (curved arrow), and yellow tissue (arrowhead) consistent with fat. (E) Photomicrograph (original magnification, ×40; hematoxylin-eosin stain) shows loose fibromyxoid stroma (asterisk) with spindle cells, and small thin-walled blood vessels. Focal mucosal ulceration (arrow) with granulation tissue also is present.

mesenchymal component histologically. These include fibromas, lipomas, fibrolipomas, fibromyxomas, and fibroepithelial polyps. These tumors contain a mixture of fibrous, vascular, and adipose tissue, which are covered by squamous epithelium. They are found most commonly as pedunculated intraluminal masses in the cervical esophagus, attached by a pedicle near the level of the cricopharyngeus.[8] Most of these polyps are 7 cm or longer at the time of presentation, and they can extend as far as 20 cm into the distal esophagus, occasionally traversing the gastroesophageal junction to enter the gastric fundus.[45] It has been theorized that these tumors gradually elongate over a period of years as the result of esophageal peristalsis pulling on them.[46] Gross pathology demonstrates a white myxoid appearance mixed with yellow adipose tissue, with microscopic examination revealing varying amounts of adipose tissue and loose or dense fibrovascular tissue, covered by normal squamous epithelium. Their cross-sectional appearance largely depends on the proportions of fat and fibrous tissue. A heterogeneous appearance from areas of fat attenuation, hyperechogenicity, or high T1 signal from adipose tissue, mixed with areas of soft tissue attenuation, hypoechogenicity, or low T1 signal from fibrovascular tissue, on CT, ultrasound, and MR imaging, respectively, is most common (**Fig. 7**).[47] Although malignant degeneration is thought to be extremely rare, removal is recommended due to their progressive and eventually debilitating nature.[7]

## SUMMARY

The imaging appearance of esophageal neoplasms and tumor-like conditions, such as fibrovascular polyps, is driven by the pathology of these tumors. The locations of tumors within the esophageal wall, along the length of the esophagus, and relative to the lumen of the esophagus are key reporting elements at initial imaging diagnosis. Although pathologic diagnosis is necessary in almost all cases, a modern clinical imager must be aware of what pathologic and imaging features drive clinical management and prognosis.

## DISCLOSURE

J.P. Lichtenberger—Author, Elsevier. A.R. Dulberger—The opinions and assertions contained herein are the private views of the authors and are not to be construed as official nor as representing the views of the Departments of the Army, Navy, Air Force, or Defense.

## REFERENCES

1. Oesophageal cancer statistics. World Cancer Research Fund. 2019. Available at: https://www.wcrf.org/dietandcancer/cancer-trends/oesophageal-cancer-statistics. Accessed May 21, 2020.
2. Siegel RL, Miller KD, Jemal A. Cancer statistics, 2020. CA Cancer J Clin 2020;70(1):7–30.
3. Rustgi AK, El-Serag HB. Esophageal carcinoma. N Engl J Med 2014;371(26):2499–509.
4. Jemal A, Bray F, Center MM, et al. Global cancer statistics. CA Cancer J Clin 2011;61(2):69–90.
5. Torre LA, Siegel RL, Ward EM, et al. Global cancer incidence and mortality rates and trends–an update. Cancer Epidemiol Biomarkers Prev 2016;25(1):16–27.
6. Abnet CC, Arnold M, Wei WQ. Epidemiology of esophageal squamous cell carcinoma. Gastroenterology 2018;154(2):360–73.
7. Levine MS. In: Gore MR, Levine MS, editors. Textbook of gastrointestinal radiology. 4th edition. Philadelphia: Saunders; 2015. p. 350–411.
8. Lewis RB, Mehrotra AK, Rodriguez P, et al. From the radiologic pathology archives: esophageal neoplasms: radiologic-pathologic correlation. Radiographics 2013;33(4):1083–108.
9. Mutrie CJ, Donahue DM, Wain JC, et al. Esophageal leiomyoma: a 40-year experience. Ann Thorac Surg 2005;79(4):1122–5.
10. Hofstetter WL. Esophageal carcinoma. In: Feig BW, editor. MD Anderson surgical Oncological Handbook. 6th ediiton. Philadelphia: Elsevier; 2019. p. 220–34.
11. Hong SJ, Kim TJ, Nam KB, et al. New TNM staging system for esophageal cancer: what chest radiologists need to know. Radiographics 2014;34(6):1722–40.
12. Glickman JO RD. Epithelial neoplasms of the esophagus. In: Odze RDG JR, editor. Surgical Pathology of the GI tract, liver, biliary tract and pancreas. 3rd ediiton. Philadelphia: Saunders/Elsevier; 2015. p. 674–706.
13. Brown IF S, Kawachi H, Lam AK, et al. Oesophageal squamous cell carcinoma NOS. In: Nagtegaal ID, Odze RD, Klimstra D, et al, editors. WHO classification of tumors. Digestive system tumors, vol. 76, 5th edition. Switzerland: IARC; 2019. p. 48–53.
14. Kato H, Momma K, Yoshida M. Early esophageal cancer: radiologic estimation of invasion into the muscularis mucosae. Abdom Imaging 2003;28(4):464–9.
15. Rice TW, Ishwaran H, Blackstone EH, et al. Recommendations for clinical staging (cTNM) of cancer of the esophagus and esophagogastric junction for the 8th edition AJCC/UICC staging manuals. Dis Esophagus 2016;29(8):913–9.
16. Levine MS. Benign tumors of the esophagus: radiologic evaluation. Semin Thorac Cardiovasc Surg 2003;15(1):9–19.

17. Boland GWL. Esophagus. In: Boland GWL, Halpert RD, editors. Gastrointestinal imaging : the requisites. 4th edition. Philadelphia: Saunders/Elsevier; 2014. p. 1–38.

18. Lee SS, Ha HK, Byun JH, et al. Superficial esophageal cancer: esophagographic findings correlated with histopathologic findings. Radiology 2005; 236(2):535–44.

19. Kim TJ, Kim HY, Lee KW, et al. Multimodality assessment of esophageal cancer: preoperative staging and monitoring of response to therapy. Radiographics 2009;29(2):403–21.

20. Botet JF, Lightdale CJ, Zauber AG, et al. Preoperative staging of esophageal cancer: comparison of endoscopic US and dynamic CT. Radiology 1991; 181(2):419–25.

21. Jiang C, Chen Y, Zhu Y, et al. Systematic review and meta-analysis of the accuracy of 18F-FDG PET/CT for detection of regional lymph node metastasis in esophageal squamous cell carcinoma. J Thorac Dis 2018;10(11):6066–76.

22. Cerfolio RJ, Bryant AS, Ohja B, et al. The accuracy of endoscopic ultrasonography with fine-needle aspiration, integrated positron emission tomography with computed tomography, and computed tomography in restaging patients with esophageal cancer after neoadjuvant chemoradiotherapy. J Thorac Cardiovasc Surg 2005;129(6):1232–41.

23. van Heijl M, Omloo JM, van Berge Henegouwen MI, et al. Fluorodeoxyglucose positron emission tomography for evaluating early response during neoadjuvant chemoradiotherapy in patients with potentially curable esophageal cancer. Ann Surg 2011;253(1):56–63.

24. Filicori F, Swanström LL. Management of esophageal cancer. In: Cameron JL, Cameron AM, editors. Current surgical therapy. 13th edition. Philadelphia: Elsevier; 2020. p. 53–63.

25. Little AG, Lerut AE, Harpole DH, et al. The Society of Thoracic Surgeons practice guidelines on the role of multimodality treatment for cancer of the esophagus and gastroesophageal junction. Ann Thorac Surg 2014;98(5):1880–5.

26. Fisher OL, RVN. Epidemiology of Barrett esophagus and risk factors for progression. In: Yeo C, editor. Shackelford's surgery of the alimentary tract. 8th edition. Philadelphia: Lippincott Williams & Wilkins; 2019. p. 323–38.

27. Siewert JR, Stein HJ, Feith M, et al. Histologic tumor type is an independent prognostic parameter in esophageal cancer: lessons from more than 1,000 consecutive resections at a single center in the Western world. Ann Surg 2001;234(3):360–7 [discussion: 368–9].

28. Yin F, Gonzaolo DH, Lai J, et al. Histopathology of Barrett's esophagus and early-stage esophageal adenocarcinoma: an updated review. Gastroentest Disord 2019;1:147–63.

29. Montgomery E. Tumors of the esophagus. In: Iacobuzio-Donahue CA, Montgomery E, editors. Gastrointestinal and liver pathology. 2nd edition. Philadelphia: Saunders/Elsevier; 2012. p. 35–64.

30. Stahl A, Ott K, Weber WA, et al. FDG PET imaging of locally advanced gastric carcinomas: correlation with endoscopic and histopathological findings. Eur J Nucl Med Mol Imaging 2003;30(2):288–95.

31. Bang YJ, Van Cutsem E, Feyereislova A, et al. Trastuzumab in combination with chemotherapy versus chemotherapy alone for treatment of HER2-positive advanced gastric or gastro-oesophageal junction cancer (ToGA): a phase 3, open-label, randomised controlled trial. Lancet 2010;376(9742):687–97.

32. Seremetis MG, Lyons WS, deGuzman VC, et al. Leiomyomata of the esophagus. An analysis of 838 cases. Cancer 1976;38(5):2166–77.

33. Dry SM, Kumarasinghe MP. Leiomyoma. In: Nagtegaal ID, Odze RD, Klimstra D, et al, editors. The 2019 WHO classification of tumours of the digestive system. vol. 76. Lyon (France): International Agency for Research on Cancer, World Health Organization; 2019. p. 182–8.

34. Yang PS, Lee KS, Lee SJ, et al. Esophageal leiomyoma: radiologic findings in 12 patients. Korean J Radiol 2001;2(3):132–7.

35. Iannicelli E, Sapori A, Panzuto F, et al. Oesophageal GIST: MDCT findings of two cases and review of the literature. J Gastrointest Cancer 2012;43(3):481–5.

36. Miettinen M, Sarlomo-Rikala M, Sobin LH, et al. Esophageal stromal tumors: a clinicopathologic, immunohistochemical, and molecular genetic study of 17 cases and comparison with esophageal leiomyomas and leiomyosarcomas. Am J Surg Pathol 2000;24(2):211–22.

37. Rocco G, Trastek VF, Deschamps C, et al. Leiomyosarcoma of the esophagus: results of surgical treatment. Ann Thorac Surg 1998;66(3):894–6 [discussion: 897].

38. Wolfel DA. Leiomyosarcoma of the esophagus. Am J Roentgenol Radium Ther Nucl Med 1963;89:127–31.

39. Graham RP, Yasir S, Fritchie KJ, et al. Polypoid fibroadipose tumors of the esophagus: 'giant fibrovascular polyp' or liposarcoma? A clinicopathological and molecular cytogenetic study of 13 cases. Mod Pathol 2018;31(2):337–42.

40. Hilal L, Barada K, Mukherji D, et al. Gastrointestinal (GI) leiomyosarcoma (LMS) case series and review on diagnosis, management, and prognosis. Med Oncol 2016;33(2):20.

41. Levine MS, Buck JL, Pantongrag-Brown L, et al. Leiomyosarcoma of the esophagus: radiographic findings in 10 patients. AJR Am J Roentgenol 1996;167(1):27–32.

42. Pesarini AC, Ernst H, Ell C, et al. [Leiomyosarcoma of the esophagus. Clinical aspects, diagnosis and therapy based on an individual case]. Med Klin (Munich) 1997;92(4):234–40.

43. Winant AJ, Gollub MJ, Shia J, et al. Imaging and clinico-pathologic features of esophageal gastrointestinal stromal tumors. AJR Am J Roentgenol 2014;203(2):306–14.

44. Miettinen M, Lasota J. Gastrointestinal stromal tumors (GISTs): definition, occurrence, pathology, differential diagnosis and molecular genetics. Pol J Pathol 2003;54(1):3–24.

45. Choong CK, Meyers BF. Benign esophageal tumors: introduction, incidence, classification, and clinical features. Semin Thorac Cardiovasc Surg 2003; 15(1):3–8.

46. Tucker HJ, Snape WJ Jr, Cohen S. Achalasia secondary to carcinoma: manometric and clinical features. Ann Intern Med 1978;89(3):315–8.

47. Levine MS, Buck JL, Pantongrag-Brown L, et al. Fibrovascular polyps of the esophagus: clinical, radiographic, and pathologic findings in 16 patients. AJR Am J Roentgenol 1996;166(4):781–7.

# Esophageal Cancer
## Tumor-Node-Metastasis Staging

Sonia L. Betancourt-Cuellar, MD[a],*, Marcelo F.K. Benveniste, MD[a], Diana P. Palacio, MD[b],
Wayne L. Hofstetter, MD[c]

## KEYWORDS

- Esophageal cancer • TNM staging system • Endoscopic ultrasound • Computed tomography
- FDG positron emission tomography/computed tomography

## KEY POINTS

- Squamous cell carcinoma and adenocarcinoma represent more than 90% of cases of esophageal cancer, the latter of which is the most prevalent histologic subtype in North America.
- The most commonly used scheme for staging esophageal cancer is the eighth edition of the American Joint Committee on Cancer/The International Union for Cancer Control TNM system.
- The T category ranges from Tis (high-grade dysplasia) to T4 (invasion of the primary tumor into adjacent structures).
- The N category is subdivided into the following components based on the number of involved regional lymph nodes: N1—1 to 2 lymph node metastases, N2—3 to 6 lymph node metastases, and N3—greater than 6 lymph node metastases.
- The M category includes M0 (no metastasis) and M1 (nonregional lymph nodal metastasis and distant visceral metastasis) subcategories.

## INTRODUCTION

Esophageal cancer is a relatively uncommon malignancy in the United States, although its incidence has been increasing since the 1980s. It currently ranks seventh in terms of incidence and sixth in overall mortality worldwide.[1] The 2 most common histologic types of esophageal cancer are squamous cell carcinoma (SCC) and adenocarcinoma (AC), representing more than 90% of all cases.[2] SCC accounts for more than 80% of all cases worldwide and is the predominant histologic type in less developed countries. In contrast, AC represents more than 60% of all cases in North American, Australia, and Europe.[3,4]

The treatment of esophageal cancer is stage-specific in order to ensure the best possible clinical outcomes. The treatment plan typically includes surgical resection for early disease, multimodality treatment with neoadjuvant chemotherapy, or combined chemoradiotherapy followed by surgery for patients with locally advanced cancer and systemic therapy for patients with metastatic disease. Accordingly, accurate pretreatment staging is important to ensure the development of appropriate treatment plans. The most commonly used staging for esophageal cancer is the eighth edition of the American Joint Committee on Cancer (AJCC)/The international Union for Cancer Control (UICC) TNM system. TNM staging includes determination of the depth of local invasion by the primary tumor (T), the presence and number of regional lymph nodes involved (N), and the presence or absence of distant metastasis (M). Because of differences in epidemiology, pathogenesis, location, and

[a] Thoracic Imaging Department, The University of Texas MD Anderson Cancer Center, 1515 Holcombe Boulevard, Unit 1478, Houston, TX 77030-4009, USA; [b] Department of Medical Imaging, The University of Arizona - Banner Medical Center, 1501 North Campbell Avenue, PO BOX 245067, Tucson, AZ 85724, USA; [c] Cardiothoracic Department, The University of Texas MD Anderson Cancer Center, 1515 Holcombe Boulevard, Unit 1489, Houston, TX 77030-4009, USA
* Corresponding author. The University of Texas MD Anderson Cancer Center, 1515 Holcombe Boulevard, Unit 1478, Houston, TX 77030-4009.
E-mail address: Slbetancourt@mdanderson.org

Radiol Clin N Am 59 (2021) 219–229
https://doi.org/10.1016/j.rcl.2020.11.008
0033-8389/21/© 2020 Elsevier Inc. All rights reserved.

outcomes of the major histologic subtypes, TNM staging is separate for AC and SCC and takes into account the differences in prognosis between clinically and pathologically staged patients. In this regard, clinical (cTNM) staging before treatment and pathologic (pTNM) staging after surgical resection are used. The eighth edition of the TNM system also includes an additional stage grouping for patients who have undergone neoadjuvant therapy and surgical resection (ypTNM).[4-6]

### Tumor-Node-Metastasis Staging System

Categories and subcategories are used in cTNM, pTNM, and ypTNM staging.[4-6] The T category represents the primary tumor, and the subcategories describe the depth of local invasion (T1–T4). Lymph node metastasis is designated by the N category, and the subcategories (N0–N3) describe the number of regional lymph nodes. The M category represents distant metastatic disease and includes subcategories describing its absence (M0) or presence (M1) (**Fig. 1**). Nonanatomic categories comprise histologic cell type, grade of differentiation (G), and location (L) of the primary tumor. Categories G and L are used only for pTNM. These anatomic and nonanatomic categories and subcategories are used to determine cTNM (based on imaging studies and histology obtained by biopsies) (**Table 1**) and pTNM (**Table 2**) and ypTNM (both based on pathology of the resected specimen) (**Table 3**).

## ANATOMIC CATEGORIES
### Clinical TNM

Currently, clinical staging of patients with esophageal cancer includes multimodality evaluation using a combination of esophagogastroduodenoscopy/endoscopic ultrasound (EUS); EUS–fine-needle aspiration (FNA); computed tomography (CT) of the chest, abdomen, and pelvis; and fluorodeoxyglucose (FDG) PET/CT. CT and FDG PET/CT complement each other in the evaluation of esophageal cancer cases. Conventional contrast-enhanced CT generally provides higher-quality images, particularly of the lungs, whereas FDG PET/CT provides functional and anatomic information useful in baseline staging and the evaluation of therapeutic response.

### Primary Tumor (cT)

The esophageal wall is composed of 3 distinct layers—mucosa, submucosa, and muscularis propria. There is no serosa, and the muscularis

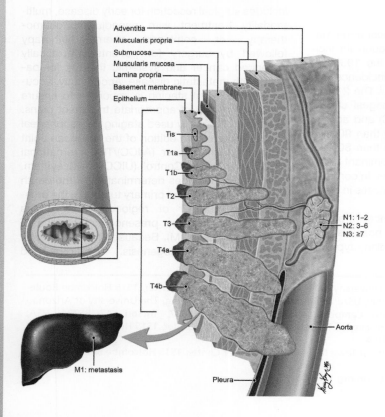

Adventitia
Muscularis propria
Submucosa
Muscularis mucosa
Lamina propria
Basement membrane
Epithelium

Tis
T1a
T1b
T2
T3
T4a
T4b

N1: 1–2
N2: 3–6
N3: ≥7

Aorta

M1: metastasis

Pleura

Fig. 1. TNM anatomic categories include the primary tumor (T), regional lymph node (N), and distant metastases (M). The T category provides information regarding the extension of tumor invasion into the esophageal wall. The N category represents regional lymph node involvement, and the M category represents metastasis to distant organ/s.

**Table 1**
**Clinical TNM stage groups**

| Clinical TNM Adenocarcinoma | | | |
|---|---|---|---|
| Stage | T | N | M |
| 0 | Tis | N0 | M0 |
| I | T1 | N0 | M0 |
| IIA | T1 | N1 | M0 |
| IIB | T2 | N0 | M0 |
| III | T2–3 | N1 | M0 |
| | T3–4a | N0–1 | M0 |
| IVA | T1–4a | N2 | M0 |
| | T4b | N0–2 | M0 |
| | T1–4 | N3 | M0 |
| IVB | Any T | Any N | M1 |
| Clinical TNM Squamous Cell Carcinoma | | | |
| Stage | T | N | M |
| 0 | Tis | N0 | M0 |
| I | T1 | N0–1 | M0 |
| II | T2 | N0–1 | M0 |
| | T3 | N0 | M0 |
| III | T3 | N1 | M0 |
| | T1–3 | N2 | M0 |
| IV | T4 | N0–2 | M0 |
| IIIA | T1–T2 | N2 | M0 |
| | T1–4 | N3 | M0 |
| IVA | T4 | N0–2 | M0 |
| IVB | Any T | Any N | M1 |

The cTNM is separate for AC and SCC, given the differences in epidemiology, pathogenesis, location and outcomes of both subtypes. cTNM is based on imaging and biopsy specimens.

**Table 2**
**Pathologic TNM stage groups**

| Pathologic TNM Adenocarcinoma | | | | |
|---|---|---|---|---|
| Stage | T | N | M | G |
| 0 | Tis | N0 | M0 | N/A |
| IA | T1a | N0 | M0 | G, X |
| IB | T1a | N0 | M0 | G2 |
| | T1b | N0 | M0 | G1–2, X |
| IC | T1 | N0 | M0 | G3 |
| | T2 | N0 | M0 | G1–2 |
| IIA | T2 | N0 | M0 | G3, X |
| IIB | T1 | N1 | M0 | Any |
| | T3 | N1 | M0 | Any |
| IIIA | T1 | N2 | M0 | Any |
| | T2 | N0–1 | M0 | Any |
| IIIB | T4a | N1–2 | M0 | Any |
| | T3 | N1 | M0 | Any |
| | T2–3 | N2 | M0 | Any |
| IVA | T4a | N2 | M0 | Any |
| | T4b | N0–2 | M0 | Any |
| | T1–4 | N3 | M0 | Any |
| | T1–4 | N0–3 | M1 | Any |

| Pathologic TNM Squamous Cell Carcinoma | | | | | |
|---|---|---|---|---|---|
| Stage | T | N | M | G | Location |
| 0 | Tis | N0 | M0 | 1, X | Any |
| IA | T1a | N0 | M0 | G1, X | Any |
| IB | T1b | N0 | M0 | G1, X | Any |
| | T1 | N0 | M0 | G2–3 | Any |
| | T2 | N0 | M0 | G1 | Any |
| IIA | T2 | N0 | M0 | G2–3, X | Any |
| | T3 | N0 | M0 | G1 | Upper/middle |
| IIB | T3 | N0 | M0 | G2–3 | Upper/middle |
| | T3 | N0 | M0 | X | Any |
| | T3 | N1 | M0 | Any | X |
| | T1 | N1 | M0 | Any | Any |
| IIIA | T1 | N2 | M0 | Any | Any |
| | T2 | N1 | M0 | Any | Any |
| IIIB | T4a | N0–1 | M0 | Any | Any |
| | T3 | N1 | M0 | Any | Any |
| | T2–3 | N2 | M1 | Any | Any |
| IVA | T4a | N2 | M0 | Any | Any |
| | T4b | N0–2 | M0 | Any | Any |
| | T1–4 | N3 | M0 | Any | Any |
| IVB | T1–4 | N0–3 | M1 | Any | Any |

The pTNM is based on pathologic findings after esophagectomy. Differences in survival profiles make it necessary to separate stage groups for AC and SCC.

propria is contiguous with the periesophageal connective tissue or adventitia. The depth of local tumor invasion (T) is determined by the involvement of each of these histologic layers and adjacent structures. The absence of a serosa facilitates local tumor invasion into the pleura, pericardium, diaphragm, and peritoneum.[7] The T subcategory ranges from Tis (high-grade dysplasia) to T4 (tumor invasion into adjacent structures) (see **Fig. 1**). Malignant cells in the epithelium confined by the basement membrane are categorized as Tis. T1 tumors are subdivided into T1a (tumor confined to the submucosa) and T1b (invasion of the submucosa) components. T2 lesions invade the muscularis propria and T3 tumors invade the adventitia. T4 lesions invade adjacent structures and are subdivided into T4a (potentially resectable invasion of the pleura, pericardium or diaphragm) and T4b (typically unresectable invasion of other

**Table 3**
**Postneoadjuvant pathologic TNM stage groups**

| Stage | T | N | M |
| --- | --- | --- | --- |
| I | T0–2 | N0 | M0 |
| II | T3 | N0 | M0 |
| IIIA | T0–2 | N1 | M0 |
| IIIB | T4a | N0 | M0 |
| III | T3 | N1–2 | M0 |
| | T0–3 | N2 | M0 |
| IVA | T4a | N1–2, X | M0 |
| | T4b | N0–2 | M0 |
| | T1–4 | N3 | M0 |
| IVB | T1–4 | N0–3 | M1 |

ypTNM is identical for both AC and SCC and is based on the pathologic review of the resected specimen in patients who have had neoadjuvant therapy.

adjacent structures, such as aorta, vertebral body or trachea) components.[4–6]

EUS is considered the imaging modality of choice for determining cT, because it provides a detailed view of the esophageal wall layers and is the most accurate modality for assessing the depth of tumor invasion, with an overall accuracy of 71% to 92%[8,9] (**Fig. 2**). Because of differences in treatment and prognosis, accurate determination of the depth of invasion is important. In this regard, Tis and T1a lesions can be treated with endoscopic resection whereas T1b tumors require esophagectomy.[9–11] The accuracy of EUS, however, in differentiating between superficial tumors (cTis, cT1a, and cT1b) is limited. A meta-analysis evaluating the accuracy of EUS in determining cTis, cT1a, and cT1b compared with specimens obtained after endoscopic and surgical resection found a cT-stage concordance of only 65%. The investigators concluded that EUS is not sufficiently accurate in differentiating high-grade dysplasia and superficial ACs.[12] In another meta-analysis, however, EUS had sensitivity of 85% and specificity of 87% for cT1a and had sensitivity and specificity of 86% for cT1b. In this study, the investigators concluded that EUS has high accuracy for staging of superficial tumors.[13] Although the literature is unclear regarding the adequacy of EUS in the staging of superficial esophageal cancer, endoscopic mucosal resection and endoscopic submucosal dissection are alternative options and provide accurate differentiation of superficial tumors as well as treatment.[14–16] The accuracy of EUS for staging cT increases in advanced tumors (cT2 and greater), with a reported accuracy of 100% in cT3.[17] EUS also can be limited, however, in the evaluation of advanced disease. In this regard, the presence of malignant strictures in 20% to 36% of these cases can mechanically preclude optimal scope placement. Additionally, the small field of view with EUS potentially can limit accurate evaluation of the depth of invasion of large T4 tumors.[9,18]

CT cannot differentiate between the histologic layers of the esophageal wall and has a relatively poor sensitivity for determining cT (approximately 67%) (**Fig. 3**).[19] CT is the most accurate imaging modality, however, for identifying the invasion of adjacent structures (cT4). The loss of the fat plane between the tumor and adjacent structures in the mediastinum is highly suggestive of local invasion. Similarly, pleural or pericardial invasion is likely when there is loss of the fat plane between the tumor and the pleura/pericardium and the presence of an effusion and/or thickening.[18] Aortic invasion is suggested if there is an area of contact between

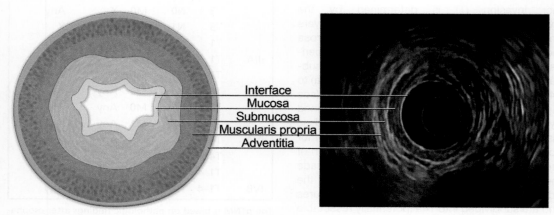

Interface
Mucosa
Submucosa
Muscularis propria
Adventitia

**Fig. 2.** EUS provides a detailed view of the esophageal wall layers and is the most accurate modality for assessing the T subcategories.

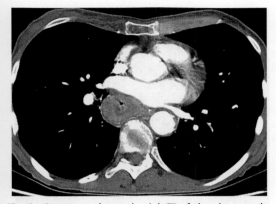

Fig. 3. Contrast-enhanced axial CT of the chest at the level of the left inferior pulmonary vein shows circumferential thickening of the esophageal wall consistent with malignancy. The precise extension of tumor invasion into the esophageal wall, however, cannot be accurately determined by CT.

the tumor and the aorta greater than 90o or if there is obliteration of the fat plane between the esophagus, aorta, and spine adjacent to the tumor.[20,21] Gross invasion of adjacent structures, including extension of the primary tumor into the lumen of the trachea, local destruction of an adjacent vertebral body, and extension of the primary malignancy, into the spinal canal are diagnostic of cT4 (Fig. 4).[22,23]

Similar to CT, the determination of the cT by FDG PET/CT is limited by poor spatial resolution. Increased FDG in the primary tumor, however, can allow detection and localization of those tumors that are not visualized anatomically. Although superficial esophageal cancer confined

to the mucosa (cT1) typically is not visualized due to tumors having volumes below the resolution of FDG PET/CT, visualization increases as cT stage increases. In a study by Kato and colleagues,[24] 43% of T1 tumors, 83% of T2 tumors, 97% of T3 tumors, and 100% of T4 tumors were detected on PET imaging due to increased FDG uptake. Focal FDG uptake in the esophagus also can occur secondary to additional factors, such as esophagitis or mucosal ulceration.[14] Another cause of false-positive FDG uptake in the esophagus is inflammation after endoscopic biopsy of the mucosa.[25] For these reasons, focal increased FDG uptake in the esophagus should be correlated with the recent clinical history and findings at endoscopy.

## Regional Lymph Nodes (cN)

The cN subcategory ranges from N0 to N3 and describes the number of regional lymph node metastases.[6] Regional lymph nodes are defined as any periesophageal lymph node from the upper esophageal sphincter to the celiac axis.[26] These include extrathoracic lymph nodes in the lower cervical periesophageal region, periesophageal intrathoracic lymph nodes, bilateral paratracheal and subcarinal nodes, diaphragmatic lymph nodes adjacent to the crura, paracardial lymph nodes, and upper abdominal lymph nodes (left gastric, common hepatic, splenic, and celiac lymph nodes). Lymph nodes outside these regions are considered distant metastatic disease.[26] Supraclavicular lymph nodes not located in the periesophageal region are considered M1 disease.

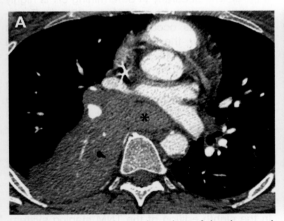
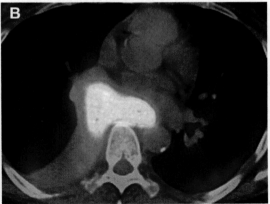

Fig. 4. (A) Contrast-enhanced axial CT of the chest at the level of the left inferior pulmonary vein shows a poorly marginated esophageal mass (asterisk) extending into the azygoesophageal recess. The mass occludes the bronchus intermedius and results in atelectasis of the right lower lobe. (B) Fused axial FDG PET/CT at the same level confirms the findings on CT. CT is the optimal modality for detecting gross extension of the primary tumor into the adjacent structures. (Courtesy of Kelly Kage, MFA, CMI, UT MD Anderson Cancer Center, Houston, TX; with permission.)

The esophagus has a rich lymph-capillary system. Most of the lymphatics are concentrated in the submucosa, although they also are present in the lamina propria. These lymphatics connect to periesophageal lymph node stations and with the thoracic duct. Lymphatic channels run radially (penetrating the esophageal wall transversally) and longitudinally (upward and downward).[27] Longitudinal lymphatic spread occurs in an expected way: tumors located in the cervical and upper thoracic esophagus drain preferentially in a cranial direction to cervical lymph nodes; tumors in the distal esophagus and gastroesophageal junction drain caudally to intra-abdominal lymph nodes; and tumors in the midthoracic esophagus can drain in either direction. Lymphatic spread is not limited, however, to these pathways. For instance, lymph node metastases along the recurrent laryngeal nerves in the neck still can occur with distal esophageal tumors.[27] Furthermore, because of the rich submucosal lymphatic plexus, metastases to distant lymph node stations can occur while bypassing regional lymph nodes. Such skip metastases are found in 10% to 20% of resected tumors.[28]

The number of involved lymph nodes has been shown to have an influence on survival, and this is reflected in the subdivision of the N category into N1 (1–2 lymph nodes involved), N2 (3–6 lymph nodes involved), and N3 (>6 lymph nodes involved) subcategories (see **Fig. 1**).[26] An important consideration is that the probability of lymph node metastases increases with greater local tumor invasion. For instances, lymph node metastases occur in up to 35% of T1b patients and up to 80% of T3 patients.[29,30]

EUS has been reported as an accurate imaging modality for determining cN. EUS assesses the size, shape, and the echogenicity pattern of the lymph nodes and is useful in determining the presence of metastasis. For instance, a rounded lymph node greater than 1 cm in short-axis diameter with well-demarcated borders and central hypoechoic area (indicating loss of the fatty hilum) is strongly suggestive of nodal disease[31] (**Fig. 5**). Because EUS and EUS-FNA have sensitivities of 85% and 97%, respectively, the AJCC strongly recommends that the latter be performed for accurate cN staging.[6] EUS-FNA diagnosis of metastasis in lymph nodes adjacent to the primary malignancy can be limited due to the passage of the biopsy needle through the primary malignancy, which can result in contamination and false-positive results.[32]

CT has a relatively low diagnostic performance for the identification of lymph node metastasis, with reported sensitivity of 50% and specificity of

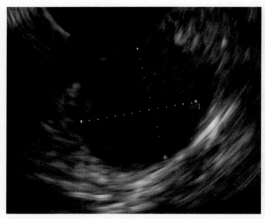

Fig. 5. EUS shows a rounded lymph node with well-defined borders and hypoechogenicity, findings suspicious for lymph node metastasis, the presence of which was confirmed by FNA biopsy.

83% when using a criteria of greater than 1 cm in short-axis diameter.[33] False-negative and false positive results occur because normal-sized lymph nodes can have microscopic metastatic disease that cannot be identified by CT, and inflammatory/infectious processes can result in hyperplasia and enlarged lymph nodes, respectively.[34] Another potential limitation of CT is in the evaluation of lymph nodes abutting or in close proximity to the primary tumor. These lymph nodes can be difficult to separate from the primary tumor and cN can be difficult to determine accurately.[31]

FDG PET/CT combines anatomic and metabolic activity in detecting lymph node metastasis (**Fig. 6**). The accuracy in determining cN is highly variable, ranging from 35% to 90%.[35] False-negative results occur because of microscopic disease below the resolution of PET/CT, and false-positive results occur in inflammatory or reactive lymph nodes. Additionally, it can be difficult to differentiate peritumoral lymph nodes from the primary tumor because intense FDG uptake by the tumor can obscure the adjacent lymph nodes. Because the reported FDG PET/CT sensitivity for cN ranges from 43% to 70% and the specificity from 76% to 95%, the role of PET/CT is limited in the evaluation of cN.[33]

## Distant Metastases (cM)

In the eighth edition of the TNM staging system, the M category is subcategorized as M0 (indicating the absence of metastasis) and M1 (representing the presence of distant metastasis). Distant metastases occur in 18% to 30% of patients at the time of presentation and are an

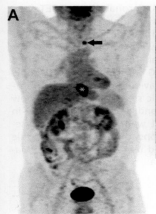
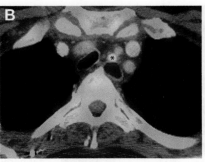

Fig. 6. (A) Coronal WB–FDG PET shows increased FDG uptake within the distal esophagus (asterisk) consistent with esophageal cancer and a smaller focus of increased FDG uptake more cephalad in the mediastinum (arrow). (B) Fused axial FDG PET/CT shows increased FDG uptake in a mediastinal lymph node (asterisk) adjacent to the esophagus suspicious for lymph node disease. cN1 was confirmed by EUS-FNA biopsy.

important factor in determining resectability.[36] The risk of hematogenous spread of the primary tumor increases with advanced local tumor invasion and lymph node involvement but also can occur early with small primary tumors and no apparent nodal metastases. The most common sites of distant metastasis include nonregional lymph nodes, liver, bone, lung, and adrenal glands.[37] Metastases in unusual sites (brain, skeletal muscle, subcutaneous fat, and thyroid gland) are considerations and occur in up to 7.7% of patients.[18,38]

CT has a reported sensitivity of 66% to 81% for the identification of distant metastases and is the ideal imaging modality detecting pulmonary metastases. A diagnostic CT using breath-hold techniques is the optimal modality to detect small lung metastases. In this regard, the imaged lungs on FDG PET/CT typically are suboptimal because they often are acquired while a patient is breathing or during partial breath-held inspiration. The resulting degradation of image quality can make detection of small nodules difficult, especially adjacent to the hemidiaphragms.[39,40]

FDG PET/CT is the imaging modality with the highest sensitivity and specificity for the detection of distant metastases (83.3% and 98.4%, respectively).[41] Several comparative studies have shown that FDG PET/CT is more accurate than CT in detecting distant metastases. FDG PET/CT increases the accuracy of clinical staging and can avoid futile surgery in patients considered for resection.[41,42] Changes in stage and treatment have been reported in approximately 30% of patients after performing FDG PET/CT imaging. In addition, synchronous tumors have been identified in 2% of patients on FDG PET/CT.[43] The high sensitivity and specificity of FDG PET/CT over other imaging modalities for the detection of distant metastases make it important in the

staging of patients with newly diagnosed esophageal cancer. Because the detection of a metastasis has a major impact on clinical management, cytologic or histopathologic confirmation of a suspected lesions identified on FDG PET/CT is strongly recommended (Fig. 7).

Early studies showed poor performance of MR imaging in the evaluation of cT and cN, mainly due to technical issues resulting in image quality degradation (swallowing, respiratory, and cardiac motion). In addition, long scan times historically have prevented more widespread use of MR imaging. Recently, studies combining T2-weighted sequences and diffusion-weighted imaging (DWI) have had shorter time duration and may be useful in determining cT and cN (Figs. 8 and 9). Gao and colleagues[44] reported an overall accuracy of MR imaging in determining the T category of 63.2% and of 50.1% for N category when combining T2-weighted sequences and DWI. An apparent diffusion coefficient (ADC) map can be derived from DWI to quantify the restricted diffusion and differentiate benign from malignant lesions. ADC can increase the detection of the primary malignancy and metastatic lymph nodes. Additionally, higher ADC values are associated with greater invasiveness and less differentiation of the primary tumor and worse overall patient prognosis. Whole-body (WB)–MR imaging, including DWI, has been reported to have accuracy similar to FDG PET/CT in detecting the primary tumor and lymph node and distant metastases.[45] In a recent study, WB–MR imaging and FDG PET/CT identified the primary tumor in 98% and 94% patients, respectively. The sensitivity and specificity for the identification of lymph node metastases were 30% and 100%, respectively, for WB–MR imaging and 27% and 100%, respectively, for FDG PET/CT. In 2 of the 49 patients, distant metastases were identified

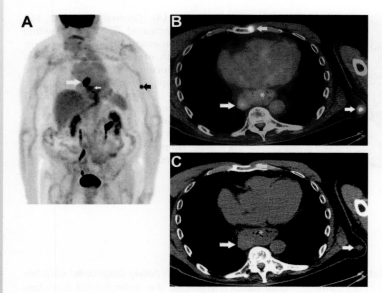

**Fig. 7.** (*A*) Coronal WB–FDG PET demonstrates multiple regions of focal increased FDG uptake in the mediastinum (*white arrows*) and the left chest wall (*black arrow*). (*B*) Fused axial FDG PET/CT and (*C*) CT show the FDG-avid primary tumor (*large arrow*), lytic sternal metastasis (*yellow arrow*), and a soft tissue nodule in the chest wall (*short arrow*). Subsequent biopsy of the chest wall nodule confirmed metastatic disease. *, hiatal hernia.

by both modalities. High-resolution (1-mm slice thickness), delayed-phase MR imaging can be used in conjunction with conventional MR imaging to further evaluate the primary tumor and has an accuracy range of 89% to 96% in determining the T subcategories.[46] A potential limitation of this technique, however, is that the small field of view can result in incomplete evaluation of large or multifocal tumors.

The potential of FDG PET/MR imaging in the preoperative staging of esophageal carcinoma has been evaluated. Lee and colleagues[45] compared the diagnostic efficacy of EUS, CT, FDG PET/CT, and FDG PET/MR imaging for the preoperative local and regional staging of esophageal cancer. For T subcategory assessment, EUS showed the highest accuracy followed by FDG PET/MR imaging and CT (86.7%, 66.7%, and 33.3%, respectively). For the N subcategory, FDG PET/MR imaging showed the highest diagnostic accuracy followed by EUS, FDG PET/CT, and CT (83%, 75%, 66.7%, and 50%,

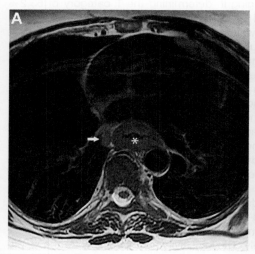
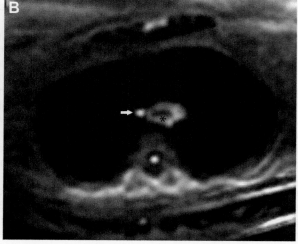

**Fig. 8.** (*A*) Axial T2-weighted MR image shows diffuse thickening of the distal esophagus consistent with a primary malignancy (*asterisk*). There is an adjacent enlarged lymph node (*arrow*) suspicious for lymph node metastasis. (*B*) Axial DWI at the same level shows high signal intensity within the esophageal wall (*asterisk*) and an adjacent lymph node (*arrow*), consistent with malignancy.

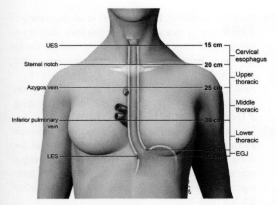

**Fig. 9.** Location of the primary esophageal cancer based on endoscopic measurements from the incisors. The esophagus is divided into 4 distinct anatomic regions. The cervical esophagus extends from the cricopharyngeus muscle to the suprasternal notch (15–20 cm from the incisors); the upper thoracic esophagus extends from the suprasternal notch to the lower border of the azygos vein (20–25 cm from the incisors); the midthoracic esophagus extends from the lower border of the azygos vein to the inferior pulmonary veins (25–30 cm from the incisors); and the lower thoracic esophagus extends from the inferior pulmonary veins to the stomach, including the intra-abdominal esophagus and the esophago-gastric junction (EGJ) (30–40 cm from the incisors). LES, lower esophageal sphincter; UES, upper esophageal sphincter. (*Courtesy of* Kelly Kage, MFA, CMI, UT MD Anderson Cancer Center, Houston, TX; with permission.)

respectively), respectively. Although FDG PET/MR imaging had an acceptable accuracy for T assessment and higher accuracy than EUS and FDG PET/CT for prediction of the N subcategory, improvements in FDG PET/MR imaging are required for it to become a routine modality in cTNM determination.

## NONANATOMIC CATEGORIES
### Histologic Cell Type

SCC usually occurs in the middle or upper one-third of the esophagus whereas AC is found most commonly in the distal esophagus and esophagogastric junction. The histologic cell type affects survival of cTNM-staged patients. For example, the survival of patients with early-stage and intermediate-stage SCC is worse than those with AC. Accordingly, SCC and AC have separate stage groupings, specifically for stage I and stage II cancers[6] (see **Table 1**).

### Grade

Histologic grade (G) reflects the biologic activity of the tumor and is subcategorized as well-

differentiated (G1), moderately differentiated (G2), and poorly differentiated (G3). If the G is undifferentiated, the tumor is considered G3. Histologic G affects the survival of patients with early-stage cancers (pT1–2NOMO AC and pT2N0M0 SCC)[6] (see **Table 2**).

### Location

The location of the primary tumor optimally is determined by esophagoscopy and is divided into 4 distinct anatomic regions that are measured from the incisors during EUS. The cervical esophagus extends from the cricopharyngeus muscle to the suprasternal notch and is 15 cm to 20 cm from the incisors by endoscopy; the upper thoracic esophagus extends from the suprasternal notch to the lower border of the azygos vein and is 20 cm to 25 cm from the incisors; the midthoracic esophagus extends from the lower border of the azygos vein to the inferior pulmonary veins and is 25 cm to 30 cm from the incisors; and the lower thoracic esophagus extends from the inferior pulmonary veins to the stomach (including the intra-abdominal esophagus and the gastroesophageal junction) and is 30 cm to 40 cm from the incisors (see **Fig. 8**). ACs with an epicenter less than or equal to 2 cm into the gastric cardia are considered esophageal cancers and those with greater than 2-cm involvement of the gastric cardia are staged as gastric cancers.[6,26] The L of the primary tumor only affects outcome in patients with SCC with stage IIA and stage IIB disease (see **Table 2**).

## SUMMARY

The incidence of esophageal cancer continues to increase, and appropriate treatment requires accurate determination of the extent of disease. In this regard, the most commonly used staging for esophageal cancer is the eighth edition of the TNM staging system. Currently, clinical staging of patients with esophageal cancer includes evaluation with EUS, CT, FDG PET/CT, MR imaging, and FDG PET/MR imaging. EUS is the best modality for determining the depth of tumor invasion (cT) and the presence of regional lymph node (cN) metastasis. CT usually is performed to evaluate whether the primary tumor invades adjacent structures as well for the detection of regional and nonregional nodal metastases and distant systemic metastases. FDG PET/CT improves the accuracy of staging and is particularly useful in the preoperative assessment of patients with esophageal cancer. Knowledge of the eighth edition TNM staging system and the appropriate use of imaging are important in ensuring appropriate patient management.

## CLINICS CARE POINTS

- The most commonly used method of staging esophageal cancer is the eighth edition of the AJCC/UICC TNM system.
- The T category represents the depth of invasion of the primary tumor into the esophageal wall. The N category represents the number of regional lymph node metastasis, and the M category represents metastasis to nonregional nodes and distant organ/s.
- EUS is the best imaging modality for determining the depth of tumor invasion (cT) and the presence of regional lymph node metastasis (cN).
- CT is used to evaluate invasion of adjacent structures and to detect regional and nonregional nodal metastasis and distant systemic metastasis.
- FDG PET/CT is useful particularly in identification of distant and unusual metastasis.

## DISCLOSURE

The authors declare that there are no conflicts of interest regarding the publication of this article.

## REFERENCES

1. Bray F, Ferlay J, Soerjomataram I, et al. Global cancer statistics 2018: GLOBOCAN estimates of incidence and mortality worldwide for 36 cancers in 185 countries. CA Cancer J Clin 2018;68(6):394–424.
2. Lewis RB, Mehrotra AK, Rodriguez P, et al. From the radiologic pathology archives: esophageal neoplasms: radiologic-pathologic correlation. Radiographics 2013;33(4):1083–108.
3. Coleman HG, Xie SH, Lagergren J. The epidemiology of esophageal adenocarcinoma. Gastroenterology 2018;154(2):390–405.
4. D'Journo XB. Clinical implication of the innovations of the 8(th) edition of the TNM classification for esophageal and esophago-gastric cancer. J Thorac Dis 2018;10(Suppl 22):S2671–81.
5. Smyth EC, Lagergren J, Fitzgerald RC, et al. Oesophageal cancer. Nat Rev Dis Primers 2017;3:17048.
6. Rice TW, Patil DT, Blackstone EH. 8th edition AJCC/UICC staging of cancers of the esophagus and esophagogastric junction: application to clinical practice. Ann Cardiothorac Surg 2017;6(2):119–30.
7. Shaheen O, Ghibour A, Alsaid B. Esophageal cancer metastases to unexpected sites: a systematic review. Gastroenterol Res Pract 2017;2017:1657310.
8. Pech O, Gunter E, Dusemund F, et al. Accuracy of endoscopic ultrasound in preoperative staging of esophageal cancer: results from a referral center for early esophageal cancer. Endoscopy 2010; 42(6):456–61.
9. Krill T, Baliss M, Roark R, et al. Accuracy of endoscopic ultrasound in esophageal cancer staging. J Thorac Dis 2019;11(Suppl 12):S1602–9.
10. May A, Gossner L, Pech O, et al. Local endoscopic therapy for intraepithelial high-grade neoplasia and early adenocarcinoma in Barrett's oesophagus: acute-phase and intermediate results of a new treatment approach. Eur J Gastroenterol Hepatol 2002; 14(10):1085–91.
11. Crumley AB, Going JJ, McEwan K, et al. Endoscopic mucosal resection for gastroesophageal cancer in a U.K. population. Long-term follow-up of a consecutive series. Surg Endosc 2011;25(2):543–8.
12. Young PE, Gentry AB, Acosta RD, et al. Endoscopic ultrasound does not accurately stage early adenocarcinoma or high-grade dysplasia of the esophagus. Clin Gastroenterol Hepatol 2010;8(12):1037–41.
13. Thosani N, Singh H, Kapadia A, et al. Diagnostic accuracy of EUS in differentiating mucosal versus submucosal invasion of superficial esophageal cancers: a systematic review and meta-analysis. Gastrointest Endosc 2012;75(2):242–53.
14. Little SG, Rice TW, Bybel B, et al. Is FDG-PET indicated for superficial esophageal cancer? Eur J Cardiothorac Surg 2007;31(5):791–6.
15. Yang D, Coman RM, Kahaleh M, et al. Endoscopic submucosal dissection for Barrett's early neoplasia: a multicenter study in the United States. Gastrointest Endosc 2017;86(4):600–7.
16. Thota PN, Sada A, Sanaka MR, et al. Correlation between endoscopic forceps biopsies and endoscopic mucosal resection with endoscopic ultrasound in patients with Barrett's esophagus with high-grade dysplasia and early cancer. Surg Endosc 2017;31(3):1336–41.
17. Shimpi RA, George J, Jowell P, et al. Staging of esophageal cancer by EUS: staging accuracy revisited. Gastrointest Endosc 2007;66(3):475–82.
18. Kim TJ, Kim HY, Lee KW, et al. Multimodality assessment of esophageal cancer: preoperative staging and monitoring of response to therapy. Radiographics 2009;29(2):403–21.
19. Rasanen JV, Sihvo EI, Knuuti MJ, et al. Prospective analysis of accuracy of positron emission tomography, computed tomography, and endoscopic ultrasonography in staging of adenocarcinoma of the esophagus and the esophagogastric junction. Ann Surg Oncol 2003;10(8):954–60. Available at: https://www.ncbi.nlm.nih.gov/pubmed/14527917. Accessed Oct.
20. Picus D, Balfe DM, Koehler RE, et al. Computed tomography in the staging of esophageal carcinoma. Radiology 1983;146(2):433–8.

21. Takashima S, Takeuchi N, Shiozaki H, et al. Carcinoma of the esophagus: CT vs MR imaging in determining resectability. AJR Am J Roentgenol 1991; 156(2):297–302.

22. Kumbasar B. Carcinoma of esophagus: radiologic diagnosis and staging. Eur J Radiol 2002;42(3): 170–80.

23. Diederich S. Staging of oesophageal cancer. Cancer Imaging 2007;7 Spec(No A):S63–6.

24. Kato H, Kuwano H, Nakajima M, et al. Usefulness of positron emission tomography for assessing the response of neoadjuvant chemoradiotherapy in patients with esophageal cancer. Am J Surg 2002; 184(3):279–83. Available at: https://www.ncbi.nlm. nih.gov/pubmed/12354600. Accessed Sep.

25. Cuellar SL, Carter BW, Macapinlac HA, et al. Clinical staging of patients with early esophageal adenocarcinoma: does FDG-PET/CT have a role? J Thorac Oncol 2014;9(8):1202–6.

26. Rice TW, Ishwaran H, Ferguson MK, et al. Cancer of the esophagus and esophagogastric junction: an eighth edition staging primer. J Thorac Oncol 2017;12(1):36–42.

27. Ji X, Cai J, Chen Y, et al. Lymphatic spreading and lymphadenectomy for esophageal carcinoma. World J Gastrointest Surg 2016;8(1):90–4.

28. Prenzel KL, Bollschweiler E, Schroder W, et al. Prognostic relevance of skip metastases in esophageal cancer. Ann Thorac Surg 2010;90(5):1662–7.

29. Lerut T, Nafteux P, Moons J, et al. Three-field lymphadenectomy for carcinoma of the esophagus and gastroesophageal junction in 174 R0 resections: impact on staging, disease-free survival, and outcome: a plea for adaptation of TNM classification in upper-half esophageal carcinoma. Ann Surg 2004;240(6):962–72 [discussion 972–64].

30. Hagen JA, DeMeester SR, Peters JH, et al. Curative resection for esophageal adenocarcinoma: analysis of 100 en bloc esophagectomies. Ann Surg 2001; 234(4):520–30 [discussion 530–21].

31. Hong SJ, Kim TJ, Nam KB, et al. New TNM staging system for esophageal cancer: what chest radiologists need to know. Radiographics 2014;34(6):1722–40.

32. Wiersema MJ, Vilmann P, Giovannini M, et al. Endosonography-guided fine-needle aspiration biopsy: diagnostic accuracy and complication assessment. Gastroenterology 1997;112(4):1087–95.

33. van Vliet EP, Heijenbrok-Kal MH, Hunink MG, et al. Staging investigations for oesophageal cancer: a meta-analysis. Br J Cancer 2008;98(3):547–57.

34. Choi JY, Lee KH, Shim YM, et al. Improved detection of individual nodal involvement in squamous cell carcinoma of the esophagus by FDG PET. J Nucl Med 2000;41(5):808–15.

35. Lerut T, Flamen P, Ectors N, et al. Histopathologic validation of lymph node staging with FDG-PET scan in cancer of the esophagus and gastroesophageal junction: A prospective study based on primary surgery with extensive lymphadenectomy. Ann Surg 2000;232(6):743–52.

36. Quint LE, Hepburn LM, Francis IR, et al. Incidence and distribution of distant metastases from newly diagnosed esophageal carcinoma. Cancer 1995; 76(7):1120–5. Available at: https://www.ncbi.nlm. nih.gov/pubmed/8630886. Accessed Oct 1.

37. Flanagan FL, Dehdashti F, Siegel BA, et al. Staging of esophageal cancer with 18F-fluorodeoxyglucose positron emission tomography. AJR Am J Roentgenol 1997;168(2):417–24.

38. Bruzzi JF, Truong MT, Macapinlac H, et al. Integrated CT-PET imaging of esophageal cancer: unexpected and unusual distribution of distant organ metastases. Curr Probl Diagn Radiol 2007;36(1):21–9. Available at: https://www.ncbi.nlm.nih.gov/pubmed/ 17198889. Accessed Jan-Feb.

39. Lowe VJ, Booya F, Fletcher JG, et al. Comparison of positron emission tomography, computed tomography, and endoscopic ultrasound in the initial staging of patients with esophageal cancer. Mol Imaging Biol 2005;7(6):422–30. Available at: https://www. ncbi.nlm.nih.gov/pubmed/16270235. Accessed Nov-Dec.

40. van Vliet EP, Steyerberg EW, Eijkemans MJ, et al. Detection of distant metastases in patients with oesophageal or gastric cardia cancer: a diagnostic decision analysis. Br J Cancer 2007;97(7):868–76.

41. Purandare NC, Pramesh CS, Karimundackal G, et al. Incremental value of 18F-FDG PET/CT in therapeutic decision-making of potentially curable esophageal adenocarcinoma. Nucl Med Commun 2014;35(8):864–9.

42. Bruzzi JF, Munden RF, Truong MT, et al. PET/CT of esophageal cancer: its role in clinical management. Radiographics 2007;27(6):1635–52.

43. Barber TW, Duong CP, Leong T, et al. 18F-FDG PET/CT has a high impact on patient management and provides powerful prognostic stratification in the primary staging of esophageal cancer: a prospective study with mature survival data. J Nucl Med 2012;53(6):864–71.

44. Gao Z, Hua B, Ge X, et al. Comparison between size and stage of preoperative tumor defined by preoperative magnetic resonance imaging and postoperative specimens after radical resection of esophageal cancer. Technol Cancer Res Treat 2019;18. 1533033819876263.

45. Lee G, I H, Kim SJ, et al. Clinical implication of PET/MR imaging in preoperative esophageal cancer staging: comparison with PET/CT, endoscopic ultrasonography, and CT. J Nucl Med 2014;55(8):1242–7.

46. Wang Z, Guo J, Qin J, et al. Accuracy of 3-T MRI for Preoperative T Staging of Esophageal Cancer After Neoadjuvant Chemotherapy, With Histopathologic Correlation. AJR Am J Roentgenol 2019;212(4): 788–95.

# Cardiac Neoplasms
## Radiologic-Pathologic Correlation

John P. Lichtenberger III, MD[a],*, Brett W. Carter, MD[b], Michael A. Pavio, MD[c],
David M. Biko, MD[d]

## KEYWORDS

- Cardiac neoplasms • Cardiac tumors • Radiologic-pathologic correlation • Computed tomography
- Magnetic resonance imaging

## KEY POINTS

- Primary cardiac neoplasms are rare, and their clinical presentation may mimic more common non-neoplastic cardiac diseases.
- The varied imaging appearances of primary cardiac neoplasms can be explained by their underlying pathology.
- Primary considerations for the imaging diagnosis of primary cardiac neoplasms are location, tissue characterization, and clinical features such as age and associated syndromes.

## INTRODUCTION

Cardiac neoplasms are a diagnostic challenge on many levels. They are rare, their clinical presentation may mimic other much more common cardiac diseases, and they are at an uncommon intersection of oncologic and cardiac imaging. Despite these obstacles, it is often possible to arrive at a favored diagnosis using advanced imaging techniques and knowledge of the pathologic basis of cardiac neoplasms. As with imaging tumors elsewhere in the thorax, a foundation in the pathology of cardiac neoplasms explains an entire spectrum of imaging appearances. Furthermore, knowledge of cardiac tumors ranging from imaging appearances to epidemiology informs the diagnostic approach to these lesions and ultimately their management. This work will explore the imaging approach to cardiac neoplasms with emphasis on the most common, clinically significant tumors and the relationship between their pathology and imaging manifestations.

An epidemiologic context is the first step to arriving at a clinically relevant diagnosis or a short differential diagnosis. Primary cardiac neoplasms are rare in both autopsy series and clinical practice, with metastatic disease being 40 to 100 times more common. This difference between the incidence of primary tumors and metastatic disease may be inconsistent with the clinical experience of cardiac imagers who frequently evaluate cardiac neoplasms. However, it should be noted that most epidemiologic data are derived from autopsy series or large clinical databases in which cardiac spread may be detected in the larger context of metastatic disease but not undergo further diagnostic evaluation.

Primary cardiac neoplasms occur at an incidence of 30 per 100,000 people per year.[1,2] Approximately 80% of primary cardiac tumors are benign. The World Health Organization has classified neoplasms of the heart into either benign tumors and tumorlike lesions such as myxoma,

[a] The George Washington University Medical Faculty Associates, 900 23rd Street Northwest, Suite G 2092, Washington, DC 20037, USA; [b] Department of Thoracic Imaging, MD Anderson Cancer Center, 1515 Holcombe Boulevard, Unit 1478, Houston, TX 77030, USA; [c] Department of Radiology, Walter Reed National Military Medical Center, 4494 North Palmer Road, Bethesda, MD 20889, USA; [d] Department of Radiology, Children's Hospital of Philadelphia and University of Pennsylvania Perelman School of Medicine, 3401 Civic Center Boulevard, Philadelphia, PA 19104, USA
* Corresponding author. 900 23rd Street Northwest, Suite G 2092, Washington, DC 20037.
E-mail address: jlichtenberger@mfa.gwu.edu

Radiol Clin N Am 59 (2021) 231–242
https://doi.org/10.1016/j.rcl.2020.10.002
0033-8389/21/© 2020 Elsevier Inc. All rights reserved.

malignant lesions such as angiosarcoma, and pericardial tumors such as solitary fibrous tumors.[3] In patients older than 16 years, the most common primary cardiac neoplasms are myxomas, lipomatous tumors, and papillary fibroelastomas. In patients younger than 16 years, the most common tumors are rhabdomyomas, teratomas, fibromas, and myxomas.[1]

The most common presenting symptom of a cardiac tumor is dyspnea, but the manifestations of a neoplasm will depend on the location of the lesion and size. Even benign cardiac tumors may cause obstruction of blood flow, decreased cardiac output, arrhythmia, or heart failure, which can be fatal.[2,4] In addition, systemic manifestations such as fatigue, anorexia, and fever may also be seen.[2]

## MYXOMA
### Clinical Considerations

Cardiac myxoma is the most common benign primary cardiac neoplasm, accounting for up to 80% of all cases,[5] but only represent 10% of benign primary cardiac tumors in children.[1] Approximately 3% to 10% of cardiac myxomas are associated with Carney complex,[6] an autosomal dominant disorder characterized by pigmented lesions of the skin and mucosae, cardiac myxomas, cutaneous tumors, and multiple other endocrine and nonendocrine neoplasms. In this disorder, pituitary neoplasms lead to acromegaly and adrenocortical tumors lead to Cushing syndrome.[7] In this disorder, cardiac myxomas are responsible for 50% of the related mortality and are often found in multiple locations, in younger patients, and have a higher risk of recurrence.[6,7]

Symptoms are variable and include shortness of breath and chest pain as well as constitutional symptoms such as fever and weight loss.[5,8] Embolism may be a presenting sign of a myxoma in up to 30% of patients.[6] Myxomas within the left heart have been shown to present earlier with worse shortness of breath when compared with right heart tumors.[8]

Although they can be located in any chamber, most myxomas are located within the left atrium and originate at the interatrial septum. These lesions may have an irregular border, a pedunculated morphology, and be mobile.[5,9] The size of the tumor is related to the degree of mobility and the potential that the lesion can obstruct the atrioventricular valve.[5]

### Pathologic Features

At gross inspection, most myxomas are soft, gelatinous, or friable lesions, ranging from 2 to 11 cm in size.[10] The contour of the tumor is most often lobular and smooth but can be villiform in appearance, which is thought to be associated to thromboembolism.[6,10]

Histologically, myxomas demonstrate myxoma cells in a myxoid stroma with possible calcification and hemorrhage. These lesions may demonstrate heterotopic elements such as bone, glands, and giant cells. In addition, the use of the immunohistochemical test of PRKAR1A, a cAMP-dependent protein kinase type 1α regulatory subunit, can be used as a screening tool to evaluate for Carney complex in the setting of myxomas.[6]

### Imaging Features

Transthoracic echocardiography is the initial imaging modality of choice for the evaluation of cardiac myxomas, although findings are nonspecific. On echocardiography, a myxoma may be heterogenous or homogeneous and may have calcification.[5] Although computed tomography (CT) is not the preferred method to characterize the tumor, typical findings on a contrast-enhanced CT include a spherical or ovoid mass that is lower in attenuation than surrounding myocardium.[10] Characteristic features of a myxoma on MR imaging is T2-weighted hyperintensity, hypoperfusion on first-pass perfusion following the administration of intravenous gadolinium, and a heterogeneous appearance on delayed enhancement when compared with the myocardium (**Figs. 1** and **2**).[5,9] Gradient echo imaging may demonstrate susceptibility artifact due to hemosiderin. Parametric techniques can also be applied to characterize the mass with T1 mapping demonstrating T1 times between 1285 and 1356 msec and T2 mapping demonstrating T2 times between 76 and 270 msec at 1.5 T.[5]

### Management

Surgical resection is the treatment of choice and is associated with excellent outcomes. In one series of 95 patients, there was only a single recurrence over 5 years following excision.[11] Patients are regularly followed with transthoracic echocardiography 1 year following excision and then at 5 years.[6]

## RHABDOMYOMA
### Clinical Considerations

Rhabdomyoma is the most common primary cardiac tumor of infancy and childhood representing 60% of pediatric primary cardiac neoplasms.[12] These lesions are most often diagnosed during the first year of life or prenatally.[13] Cardiac

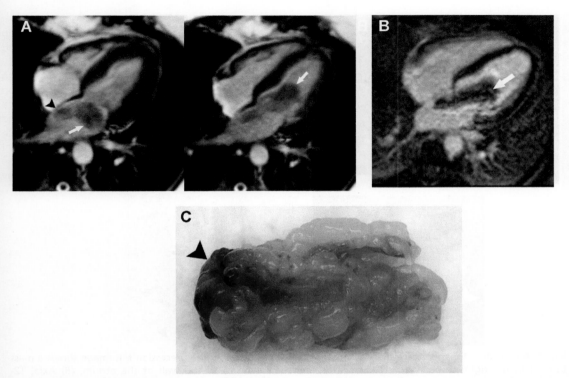

**Fig. 1.** A 35-year-old man with cardiac myxoma. (*A*) Axial SSFP MR composite image shows a mass (*arrow*) in the left atrium with stalklike attachment (*arrowhead*) to the interatrial septum. Note the prolapse of the mass across the mitral valve plane between systole (*left*) and diastole (*right*), characteristic of myxoma. (*B*) Axial late gadolinium enhancement MR image shows small foci of internal enhancement, a useful differentiating feature from thrombus. (*C*) Gross specimen shows the cut stalk (*arrowhead*) and a smooth polypoid mass. SSFP, steady-state free precession.

rhabdomyomas are associated with tuberous sclerosis in 30% to 50% of cases but also occur sporadically and rarely in association with congenital heart disease.[13,14] Tuberous sclerosis is characterized by cortical tubers and subependymal nodules within the brain, multiple retinal hamartomas, adenoma sebaceum of the skin, and periungual fibromas.[14] Rhabdomyomas may precede other sequelae of tuberous sclerosis such as skin abnormalities and neuroimaging findings by months or years.[12] Symptoms of cardiac rhabdomyomas vary and are based on the size and location of the tumor. They may be asymptomatic or result in congestive heart failure from obstruction. Arrhythmias have also been reported.[15]

Rhabdomyomas are most commonly located within the ventricles attached to the myocardium but are less commonly located in the atrioventricular groove.[9,12] They are multiple in 60% of cases, typically in the setting of tuberous sclerosis.[12]

## Pathologic Features

At gross inspection, rhabdomyomas are lobulated masses with a glistening cut surface. Sporadic

tumors tend to be larger in size than those associated with tuberous sclerosis.[13] At histology, these neoplasms tend to have large cells in relation to the myocardium with abundant glycogen. "Spider cells" are present in all tumors that have a centrally located mass of granular cytoplasm with elongated projection of myofibrils extending peripherally from the nucleus to the cell membrane.[13,16] These lesions demonstrate positive immunohistochemical staining for desmin, actin, and myoglobin.[13]

## Imaging Features

On transthoracic echocardiography, rhabdomyomas are uniformly hyperechoic in appearance (**Fig. 3**).[12] On contrast-enhanced CT, they are most often hypodense masses with little contrast enhancement.[17] On MR imaging, these tumors are homogenous in appearance, isointense to slightly hyperintense to myocardium on T1-weighted imaging, mildly hyperintense in relation to the myocardium on T2-weighted imaging, hypoenhancing on first pass perfusion, and isointense

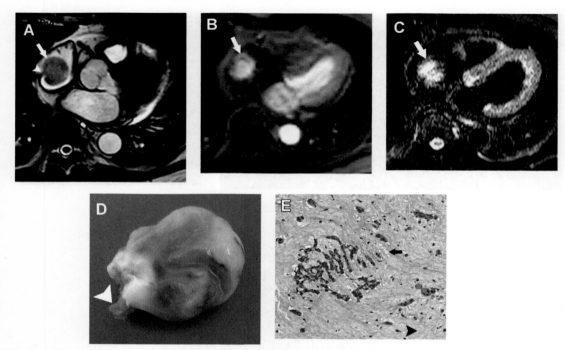

**Fig. 2.** A 62-year-old man with cardiac myxoma. (*A*) Axial steady-state free precession MR image shows a mass (*arrow*) in the right atrium with stalklike attachment (*arrowhead*) to the wall of the atrium. (*B*) Axial T2-weighted MR image shows significant hyperintensity of the mass (*arrow*), attributed to the myxoid component of these tumors. (*C*) Axial perfusion MR image in the early arterial phase shows diffuse enhancement of the mass (*arrow*), excluding thrombus as a diagnostic consideration. (*D*) Gross specimen shows the cut stalk of the mass (*arrowhead*) and a variegated white and gray tan external surface. (*E*) Photomicrograph (original magnification, 40x; hematoxylin-eosin stain) shows spindle cells without atypia (*arrowhead*) and paucicellular myxoid material (*arrow*).

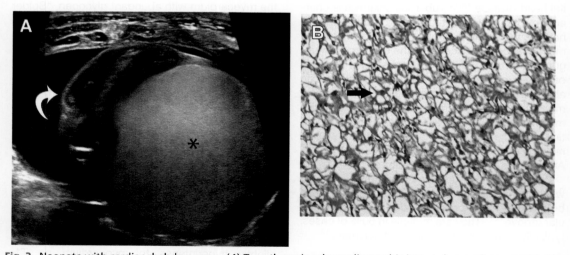

**Fig. 3.** Neonate with cardiac rhabdomyoma. (*A*) Transthoracic echocardiographic image shows a homogeneously hyperechoic mass (*asterisk*) displacing the heart to the right (*curved arrow*). (*B*) Photomicrograph (original magnification, 40x; hematoxylin-eosin stain) shows large vacuolated cells with centrally placed nucleus and myofibrils radiating to the cell membrane, "spider cells" (*arrow*).

to myocardium on myocardial delayed enhancement.[9,12]

## Management

Most rhabdomyomas spontaneously regress.[18] When there is outflow obstruction leading to heart failure or arrhythmias, surgical resection may be performed. In addition, everolimus, a mammalian target of rapamycin inhibitor, may be used as therapy.[12]

## FIBROMA
### Clinical Considerations

Cardiac fibroma is the second most common primary cardiac neoplasm of infancy and childhood after rhabdomyoma.[13] Although cases do occur in adults, greater than 80% of cardiac fibromas are in children.[19] These tumors occur more frequently in nevoid basal cell carcinoma (Gorlin) syndrome, a phakomatosis characterized by multiple basal cell carcinomas; odontogenic cysts; ocular pathology such as congenital cataracts, microphthalmia, and coloboma of the iris; and other tumors such as medulloblastoma. Two percentage of patients younger than 45 years with basal cell carcinomas have this syndrome.[20]

Patients with cardiac fibromas may be asymptomatic but may also present with arrhythmias, congestive heart failure, and sudden death believed to be secondary to distortion of the conducting system of the heart rather than infiltration.[19] The most common locations of a cardiac fibroma are the left ventricular free wall, interventricular septum, and right ventricular free wall.[21]

### Pathologic Features

At gross inspection, cardiac fibromas tend to be solitary well-demarcated white tumors ranging from 3 to 8 cm in diameter. Cut surfaces are either white, gray, or tan (**Fig. 4**). At histology, the tumor contains prominent spindle-shaped fibroblasts with a collagen matrix.[19] The collagen matrix increases with age and the amount of cellularity decreases with age.[22] Cells express alpha smooth muscle actin and do not express desmin, CD 34, or S100 protein.[19] Calcification is seen but this is more likely in older patients.[22]

### Imaging Features

Chest radiographs may show calcification in cardiac fibromas.[21] Transthoracic echocardiography is successful in identification of the mass and demonstrates mixed echogenicity. On contrast-enhanced CT, fibromas tend to enhance either homogenously or heterogeneously.[21] On MR imaging, the lesion may have a thin rim of myocardium with a heterogeneous signal intensity on both T1- and T2-weighted images. Following the administration of intravenous gadolinium, the mass demonstrates avid hyperenhancement on delayed imaging with or without decreased enhancement centrally.[9]

## Management

Surgical resection is the treatment of choice for cardiac fibromas with excellent early and late-term outcomes. If a tumor is difficult to resect due to location, subtotal resection has also been shown to result in excellent long-term survival.[23]

## HEMANGIOMA
### Clinical Considerations

Hemangiomas account for 5% to 10% of all benign cardiac neoplasms and can occur in any age group.[24] Although patients are often asymptomatic, the most common symptom is dyspnea on exertion.[25] Rarely patients may develop Kasabach-Merritt syndrome manifesting as recurrent thrombocytopenia and consumptive coagulopathy.[24] These tumors can occur in any chamber of the heart but are most common in the ventricles.[4]

### Pathologic Features

At gross inspection, hemangiomas are red and hemorrhagic.[26] On histology, there are 3 variants capillary, cavernous, and arteriovenous. The lesions are composed of a dilated mixture of mature vessels supported by fibrous connective tissue.[24]

### Imaging Features

Transthoracic echocardiography of a hemangioma reveals a solid vascular mass.[12] On contrast-enhanced CT, hemangiomas are heterogeneous masses that may contain calcifications and avidly enhance.[17] On MR imaging, hemangiomas are heterogeneous and hyperintense to myocardium on T2-weighted imaging[4] and isointense to hypointense to myocardium on T1-weighted imaging (**Fig. 5**).[25] They enhance on first pass perfusion but may have variable enhancement on myocardial delayed imaging.[9] Differentiation of hemangiomas from other vascular tumors, even malignant neoplasms such as angiosarcoma, can be difficult on MR imaging.[12]

### Management

Surgery remains the treatment of choice; however, the complication rate is higher than other neoplasms given the vascularity of hemangiomas.

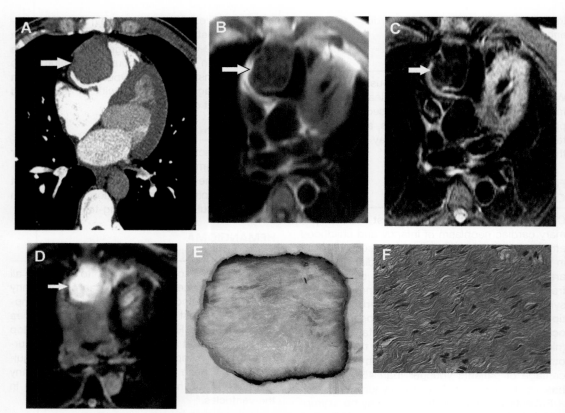

**Fig. 4.** A 45-year-old man with cardiac fibroma. (*A*) Contrast-enhanced axial CT image shows a smooth, well-circumscribed right ventricular mass (*arrow*) without pericardial effusion or evidence of local invasion. (*B*) Axial T1-weighted MR image shows the mass (*arrow*) to be uniform and slightly hypointense relative to skeletal muscle. (*C*) Axial T2-weighted MR image shows uniform hypointensity of the mass (*arrow*) without cystic components. (*D*) Axial late gadolinium enhancement MR image shows intense, diffuse enhancement (*arrow*) of the mass suggesting fibrotic tissue. (*E*) Sectioned gross specimen shows a homogeneous, whirled, white, solid cut surface. (*F*) Photomicrograph (original magnification, 40x; hematoxylin-eosin stain) shows multiple bland fibroblasts with normal appearing nuclei and no evidence of mitosis.

Preoperative coil embolization can be considered to reduce complications.[24]

## ANGIOSARCOMA
### Clinical Considerations

Cardiac angiosarcomas are the most common primary cardiac malignancy in adults with specific differentiation, accounting for 40% of cardiac sarcomas. Patients are usually younger than 65 years, peaking in the fourth to fifth decade, with a slight male preponderance of 1.3:1.[27]

Cardiac angiosarcomas occur almost exclusively in the right atrium near the atrioventricular sulcus (80%–90% of cases). Symptoms generally result from obstruction, tumor emboli, or local invasion into the myocardium and atrial free wall. A common presentation includes chest tightness, dizziness, dyspnea, and symptoms related to congestive right heart failure.

Nonspecific symptoms such as weight loss, malaise, anemia, and fatigue may also coexist. Pericardial effusion, which is diagnosed in 56% of patients, can manifest as cardiac tamponade and occurs more frequently in cardiac angiosarcomas than with other types of cardiac sarcoma due to the propensity for pericardial involvement. An insidious onset of arrythmia is frequently described in the young and often indicates myocardial invasion.[28]

These tumors are prone to local and distant metastases with the lung being the most common site. Additional areas reported include the liver, mediastinal lymph nodes, bone, adrenal glands, and spleen. Patients undergoing surgical resection interestingly demonstrate a propensity for brain metastases, thought to be due to intravascular dissemination at tumor resection and manipulation.[29]

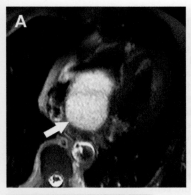
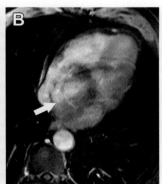
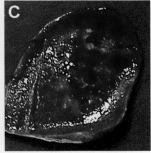
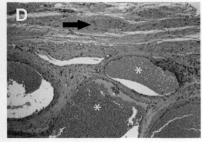

**Fig. 5.** A 71-year-old man with cardiac hemangioma. (*A*) Axial T2-weighted MR image shows a homogeneously hyperintense intracardiac mass (*arrow*) displacing the adjacent cardiac chambers. (*B*) Axial postcontrast T1-weighted MR image shows heterogeneous internal enhancement. (*C*) Sectioned gross specimen shows an encapsulated mass with red-tan, spongy fibrous tissue and maroon-red fluid. (*D*) Photomicrograph (original magnification, 40x; hematoxylin-eosin stain) shows dilated vascular channels (*asterisk*) and overlying myocardium (*arrow*).

## Pathologic Features

Cardiac angiosarcomas occur in the right atrium 80% to 90% of the time. At surgical resection, the mass typically projects into the cardiac chambers with permeative growth into the myocardium and local invasion of the pericardium, vena cava, tricuspid valve, and even the coronary arteries. Gross pathology reveals a large lobulated mass that is dark red and brown in color, reflecting its hemorrhagic and necrotic components. If pericardial invasion is present, a thickened rind of gray-black tissue is observed that is inseparable from the remainder of the tumor.[30]

Histologically, the predominant feature is multiple endothelial-lined vascular channels with branching anastomoses and sinusoids. Interspersed are densely packed populations of anaplastic spindle cells that resemble those of Kaposi sarcoma. The epithelioid variant, which is most common in the heart, is characterized by round cells with abundant cytoplasm and frequent mitoses. Immunohistochemistry can be used as an adjunct when evaluating these tumors. Staining is variable and heterogeneous, dependent on the dominant histologic pattern. Staining for CD31 is positive in more than 90% of cases but is nonspecific for cardiac angiosarcomas. Expressivity of BNH9, a monoclonal antibody against blood group–related H and Y antigens, is the most specific marker.[31]

## Imaging Features

The presentation of dyspnea and congestive heart failure typically prompts evaluation with echocardiography or coronary angiography. The sensitivity of transesophageal echocardiography for the detection of cardiac masses is 75% to 97%.[30,32] Information about tumor location, shape, size, attachment, and mobility are provided by this modality. CT, MR imaging, and fluorodeoxyglucose (FDG) PET/CT usually provide further mass characterization and metastatic evaluation.

Two morphologic types have been described on imaging. The first is that of a discrete low-attenuating mass, 6 cm in average size, with irregular boarders and a broad attachment to the myocardium, most commonly arising from the right atrial free wall (**Fig. 6**).[33,34] Cavitations may decompress and freely communicate with the cardiac chambers, spilling tumor elements into the systemic circulation. Calcifications may also be present. The extent of myocardial invasion, mass effect on the cardiac chambers, and involvement of the great vessel are also pertinent findings. The second morphologic type is a diffusely infiltrative mass inseparable from the pericardium. A

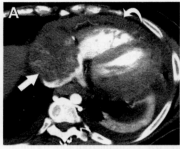
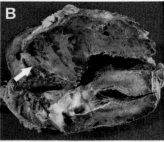
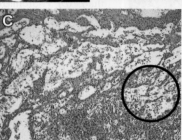

Fig. 6. A 25-year-old man with cardiac angiosarcoma. (*A*) Contrast-enhanced axial CT image shows an aggressive mass (*arrow*) centered in the right atrium with internal vascular enhancement. A pericardial effusion is present (*curved arrow*). (*B*) Sectioned gross specimen shows the mass (*arrow*) with internal dilated vessels. (*C*) Photomicrograph (original magnification, 40x; hematoxylin-eosin stain) shows a proliferation of vascular interconnected spaces (*circle*) and malignant spindle and epithelioid cells.

complex, mixed density pericardial effusion is invariably present, frequently with hemorrhagic and necrotic tumor debris. Pericardiocentesis yields a bloody aspirate that may contain malignant cells.[35]

Tumor location, tissue composition, and local invasion are often shown to better advantage on cardiac MR imaging (CMR) compared with other modalities with an additional benefit of differentiating between neoplasm and tumor mimics (such as thrombus). CMR classically demonstrates an aggressive hypervascular mass with intense heterogeneous enhancement. Intralesional flow voids, related to large tumoral vessels, are well displayed on spin echo sequences. In addition, CMR patterns can differ between the 2 morphologic subtypes. The first pattern is characterized by a heterogeneous "cauliflower"-shaped mass that is hyperintense on both T1-and T2-weighted images that indicate hemorrhagic and necrotic content. The second morphology of diffuse pericardial infiltration appears as pericardial thickening and effusion with linear contrast material occupying vascular channels, producing a "sunray" appearance on the postcontrast sequences.[33] The 2 imaging patterns may coexist in the same patient.

## Management

The prognosis for cardiac angiosarcoma is poor, due to its rarity, resistance to chemoradiotherapy, and early metastasis, which is found in 56% to 89% of cases at presentation.[36] A recent

retrospective study of 68 patients reports a median overall survival of 13 months for the entire cohort, which is shorter than that of other sarcoma subtypes. However, of those presenting with metastatic disease, the median overall survival dropped to 6 months.[27] The treatment remains controversial and is most often multidisciplinary. Surgical debulking or total resection is the mainstay, particularly in the setting of localized disease. A postsurgical survival of 1 to 60 months, with a median overall survival of 11 to 14 months, has been reported in 2 separate reviews.[27,37] In contrast, a 1-year survival of 10% is shown in patients with medical therapy alone.[38]

Surgical outcomes are further optimized with neoadjuvant chemotherapy, which uses a doxorubicin-/ifosfamide-based regimen. This regimen has been shown to extend median overall survival to 15.5 months from 12 months.[32] Most cases, however, are nonsurgical; thus, treatment depends largely on cytotoxic chemotherapy, such as anthracycline, ifosfamide, and taxanes. A recent trend combines cytotoxic and targeted drug therapies, with the latter focusing on vascular endothelial growth factor A and tyrosine kinase. For example, a trial using pazopanib combination therapy reports a median overall survival of nearly 10 months.[39]

## OTHER SARCOMAS
### Clinical Considerations

Most of the primary malignant cardiac tumors are sarcomas, accounting for greater than 90% of cases. Undifferentiated high-grade pleomorphic sarcoma (UHGPS), rhabdomyosarcoma (RS), osteosarcoma (OS), and leiomyosarcoma (LS) are discussed further. The most common of these tumors is UHGPS, previously known as malignant fibrous histiocytoma. UHGPS has a slight female predominance with a mean age of 47 years with a wide age range. RS, on the other hand, is the most common primary cardiac malignancy of childhood. A slight male predilection has been reported, and unlike other sarcomas, no chamber preference is observed. As such, clinical presentation varies. LS and OS account for less than 20% of sarcomas and typically occur in the left atrium.[40]

Presenting symptoms among cardiac sarcomas are nonspecific and include chest pain, palpitations, and embolic phenomena. Patients may also present with syncope, pneumonia, fever, arrhythmias, peripheral edema, and sudden death. Because UHGPS has a left atrial predilection, symptoms related to pulmonary congestion, mitral stenosis, and pulmonary vein obstruction can be seen.

### Pathologic Features

Cardiac sarcomas appear as large, aggressive, multifocal masses with a tendency to infiltrate multiple cardiac chambers, although generally with a left heart predilection. On gross inspection, sarcomas are described as soft, lobulated, gelatinous masses containing necrotic areas. Histologically, UHGPS is composed of undifferentiated spindle cells with frequent mitotic activity and nuclear pleomorphism, sharing histologic features with intimal sarcomas of the aorta and pulmonary artery. It often has storiform architecture with variable degrees of collagenized stroma.

### Imaging Features

Primary cardiac sarcomas are generally aggressive, heterogeneous masses that have a broad-based attachment with internal necrosis and cavitations. Violation of tissues planes is typical with associated pericardial effusions and lymphadenopathy. At CMR, these tumors exhibit heterogeneous high signal on T2-weighted imaging and low-to-intermediate signal on T1-weighted imaging with a variegated pattern of enhancement.

Location is usually the most helpful feature in suggesting a tissue diagnosis. For example, UHGPS, OS, and LS typically arise from the posterior wall of the left atrium in contradistinction to a septal origin of cardiac myxoma and a right heart location of angiosarcoma.[41] Certain mass characteristics, when present, can provide further delineation. If dense, amorphous calcifications of osteoid matrix deposition are present, OS is favored. If there is invasion of the pulmonary veins or mitral valve in a slightly younger adult patient, a diagnosis of LS can be suggested. RS presents as multiple masses always involving the myocardium with extracardiac extension common, tending to be nodular in growth rather than sheetlike.[33]

### Management

Outcomes are generally grim for cardiac sarcomas, even when detected early and aggressive therapy is used. For UHGPS, a median overall survival of 15 months (range of 11–18 months) is reported in patients following tumor surgical resection[42] but drops to 5 months in nonoperable cases. The role of chemotherapy and/or radiation therapy is controversial. Combination therapy with ifosfamide, doxorubicin, cyclophosphamide, and paclitaxel can be used with varying degrees of response. Cardiac transplantation, however, does not provide significant survival benefit.[43]

## CARDIAC LYMPHOMA
### Clinical Considerations

Primary cardiac lymphoma (PCL) is a rare extranodal lymphoma accounting for 1% to 1.5% of all primary cardiac tumors, with the majority involving the right heart. PCLs are aggressive and are usually of the non-Hodgkin type. A typical patient is an immunocompetent male adult (2:1 male to female ratio) in his 6th to 7th decade of life. The mean age is 60 years with a range of 12 to 86 years.[44] Certain subtypes occur more commonly in the immunocompromised. Posttransplant lymphoproliferative disorder, a B-cell proliferation related to Epstein-Barr virus infection, may develop mostly in lung and cardiac transplant recipients. Primary effusion lymphoma (PEL) uniquely affects patients with human immunodeficiency virus, which is associated with human herpesvirus-8 (HHV-8)/Kaposi sarcoma–associated herpesvirus.

Symptoms are variable, with dyspnea, congestive heart failure, constitutional complaints, and chest pain being the most common clinical symptoms. The anatomic location produces specific clinical syndromes. For example, right atrial lymphoma may obstruct venous inflow and cause superior vena cava syndrome, which is seen in 5% to 8% of cases.[44] Alternatively, tumor infiltration may induce arrhythmia or cause coronary artery obstruction, the latter resulting in angina. Tumor embolism and pericardial effusion with or without tamponade are also typical. Diagnosis can be made from pericardial fluid analysis, although direct endomyocardial biopsy is commonly performed.

## Pathologic Features

At gross inspection, PCLs are gray-white coalescing masses with a "fish flesh" consistency, most commonly in the right heart.[44] Most of the PCLs are of B-cell lineage and in 80% of cases are of the diffuse large B-cell lymphoma (DLBCL) type.[45] DLBCL demonstrates a uniform population of lymphoid cells on histology that express markers such as CD19, CD20, CD22, CD79a, or PAX-5, which establish a B-cell lineage. Classic type DLBCL is most commonly observed. Chronic inflammation-associated DLBCL and PEL variants are described, the former occurring in association with valve replacements and the latter occurring in association with HHV-8 infection in the immunocompromised. Burkitt lymphoma and follicular lymphoma comprise the remainder of B-cell subtypes.[46] Differentiation can be made by expressivity of CD5, CD23, and BcL-2 antigens, which are present in follicular subtype and further corroborated by c-myc gene translocations seen in Burkitt lymphoma.[44]

## Imaging Features

PCL commonly presents as a homogenously low-attenuating, hypoenhancing mass on contrast-enhanced CT, involving the right atrium or right ventricle in 92% of cases.[47] Necrosis and involvement of the cardiac valves are atypical and, if present, should invoke an alternative diagnosis such as angiosarcoma. Extension along the epicardial surface with encasement of the coronary arteries, aortic root, and great vessels is classic (Fig. 7).[33] There is often pericardial thickening and massive pericardial effusion, which can occasionally be the only imaging manifestation, particularly in the PEL subtype.[48] Stigmata of elevated right heart pressures are then assessed.

Similar to lymphoma elsewhere, PCL is highly metabolic. Although FDG PET/CT imaging is valuable in initial staging, it is usually used to monitor treatment response. Interpretation is occasionally made difficult by physiologic myocardial activity. A nodular pattern of intense radiotracer uptake (standardized uptake value >10) with a correlative mass on the CT images improves diagnostic and staging accuracy.[49]

Additional information can be obtained through CMR, specifically the assessment of tumor mobility and tumor point attachment, which is best shown on cine steady-state free precession (SSFP) imaging. SSFP also provides high-contrast resolution between tumor, myocardium, blood pool, and adjacent soft tissues. Tissue characterization is generally performed on conventional T1- and T2-weighted sequences. PCLs demonstrate signal characteristics of hypercellular tumors: hypointense on T1-weighted imaging and mildly hyperintense on T2-weighted imaging. The enhancement pattern of this tumor is variable, either homogeneous or heterogeneous. The value of postcontrast imaging is the differentiation between tumor and thrombus with thrombus demonstrating no central contrast uptake.

## Management

Treatment is often multimodal and includes surgical, medical, and radiotherapeutic approaches. Considered a systemic disease, chemotherapy is the mainstay with a regimen historically including anthracycline-containing agents, doxorubicin, vincristine, and prednisone. Combination immunotherapy with rituximab can also be used. Surgery and radiation therapy are usually performed for symptom relief.

The prognosis for both primary and secondary PCL is generally poor with a median overall survival of 63 months, reported in a recent retrospective study.[47] This is in contrast to a median overall survival of 12 months previously reported.[50]

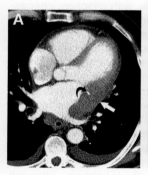
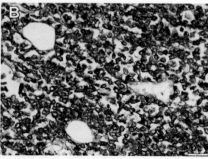

Fig. 7. A 69-year-old man with cardiac large B-cell lymphoma. (A) Contrast-enhanced axial CT image shows a mass (arrow) centered on the left atrioventricular groove, surrounding but not occluding the left circumflex coronary artery (curved arrow). (B) Photomicrograph (original magnification, 40x; CD20 stain) shows diffuse positive staining for B-cell marker CD20.

## SUMMARY

When confronted with a cardiac mass, the most important imaging considerations are the location of the tumor, the possibility of metastatic disease, and the clinical presentation. When considering the differential diagnosis for primary malignant cardiac masses, location is usually the most helpful feature. Myxomas tend to be left sided, and their overall frequency skews left-sided heart masses as more frequently benign. Cardiac lymphoma and angiosarcoma, the most common primary cardiac malignancies are predominantly right sided. Necrosis, surface enhancement ("sun-ray" appearance), and valvular involvement favor angiosarcoma, whereas homogeneity and vascular encasement favor lymphoma. Other cardiac sarcomas tend to be left sided, specifically arising from the posterior wall of the left atrium.

The pathology of primary cardiac tumors explains their varied imaging features, including calcification in OS and T2 hyperintensity in myxoma. Integrating the imaging and pathologic features of cardiac tumors furthers our understanding of the spectrum of appearances of these tumors and improves the clinical imager's ability to confidently make a diagnosis.

## DISCLOSURE

Author, Elsevier.

## REFERENCES

1. Poterucha TJ, Kochav J, O'Connor DS, et al. Cardiac Tumors: Clinical Presentation, Diagnosis, and Management. Curr Treat Options Oncol 2019; 20(8):66.

2. Rahouma M, Arisha MJ, Elmously A, et al. Cardiac tumors prevalence and mortality: A systematic review and meta-analysis. Int J Surg 2020;76:178–89.

3. Travis WD, Brambilla E, Nicholson AG, et al. The 2015 World Health Organization Classification of Lung Tumors: Impact of Genetic, Clinical and Radiologic Advances Since the 2004 Classification. J Thorac Oncol 2015;10(9):1243–60.

4. Lichtenberger JP 3rd, Dulberger AR, Gonzales PE, et al. MR Imaging of Cardiac Masses. Top Magn Reson Imaging 2018;27(2):103–11.

5. Colin GC, Gerber BL, Amzulescu M, et al. Cardiac myxoma: a contemporary multimodality imaging review. Int J Cardiovasc Imaging 2018;34(11): 1789–808.

6. Maleszewski JJ, Anavekar NS, Moynihan TJ, et al. Pathology, imaging, and treatment of cardiac tumours. Nat Rev Cardiol 2017;14(9):536–49.

7. Correa R, Salpea P, Stratakis CA. Carney complex: an update. Eur J Endocrinol 2015;173(4):M85–97.

8. Khan H, Chaubey S, Uzzaman MM, et al. Clinical presentation of atrial myxomas does it differ in left or right sided tumor? Int J Health Sci (Qassim) 2018;12(1):59–63.

9. Beroukhim RS, Prakash A, Buechel ER, et al. Characterization of cardiac tumors in children by cardiovascular magnetic resonance imaging: a multicenter experience. J Am Coll Cardiol 2011;58(10):1044–54.

10. Grebenc ML, Rosado-de-Christenson ML, Green CE, et al. Cardiac myxoma: imaging features in 83 patients. Radiographics 2002;22(3):673–89.

11. Garatti A, Nano G, Canziani A, et al. Surgical excision of cardiac myxomas: twenty years experience at a single institution. Ann Thorac Surg 2012;93(3): 825–31.

12. Tao TY, Yahyavi-Firouz-Abadi N, Singh GK, et al. Pediatric cardiac tumors: clinical and imaging features. Radiographics 2014;34(4):1031–46.

13. Freedom RM, Lee KJ, MacDonald C, et al. Selected aspects of cardiac tumors in infancy and childhood. Pediatr Cardiol 2000;21(4):299–316.

14. Harding CO, Pagon RA. Incidence of tuberous sclerosis in patients with cardiac rhabdomyoma. Am J Med Genet 1990;37(4):443–6.

15. Smythe JF, Dyck JD, Smallhorn JF, et al. Natural history of cardiac rhabdomyoma in infancy and childhood. Am J Cardiol 1990;66(17):1247–9.

16. Fenoglio JJ Jr, MCAllister HA Jr, Ferrans VJ. Cardiac rhabdomyoma: a clinicopathologic and electron microscopic study. Am J Cardiol 1976;38(2): 241–51.

17. Liddy S, McQuade C, Walsh KP, et al. The Assessment of Cardiac Masses by Cardiac CT and CMR Including Pre-op 3D Reconstruction and Planning. Curr Cardiol Rep 2019;21(9):103.

18. Wu SS, Collins MH, de Chadarevian JP. Study of the regression process in cardiac rhabdomyomas. Pediatr Dev Pathol 2002;5(1):29–36.

19. Gotlieb AI. Cardiac fibromas. Semin Diagn Pathol 2008;25(1):17–9.

20. Gorlin RJ. Nevoid basal cell carcinoma (Gorlin) syndrome. Genet Med 2004;6(6):530–9.

21. Grunau GL, Leipsic JA, Sellers SL, et al. Cardiac Fibroma in an Adult AIRP Best Cases in Radiologic-Pathologic Correlation. Radiographics 2018;38(4): 1022–2026.

22. Burke AP, Rosado-de-Christenson M, Templeton PA, et al. Cardiac fibroma: clinicopathologic correlates and surgical treatment. J Thorac Cardiovasc Surg 1994;108(5):862–70.

23. Cho JM, Danielson GK, Puga FJ, et al. Surgical resection of ventricular cardiac fibromas: early and late results. Ann Thorac Surg 2003;76(6):1929–34.

24. Maleszewski JJ, Bois MC, Bois JP, et al. Neoplasia and the Heart: Pathological Review of Effects With Clinical and Radiological Correlation. J Am Coll Cardiol 2018;72(2):202–27.

25. Sparrow PJ, Kurian JB, Jones TR, et al. MR imaging of cardiac tumors. Radiographics 2005;25(5): 1255–76.

26. Bloor CM, O'Rourke RA. Cardiac tumors: clinical presentation and pathologic correlations. Curr Probl Cardiol 1984;9(6):7–48.

27. Zhang C, Huang C, Zhang X, et al. Clinical characteristics associated with primary cardiac angiosarcoma outcomes: a surveillance, epidemiology and end result analysis. Eur J Med Res 2019;24(1):29.

28. Hamidi M, Moody JS, Weigel TL, et al. Primary cardiac sarcoma. Ann Thorac Surg 2010;90(1):176–81.

29. Butany J, Yu W. Cardiac angiosarcoma: two cases and a review of the literature. Can J Cardiol 2000; 16(2):197–205.

30. Patel SD, Peterson A, Bartczak A, et al. Primary cardiac angiosarcoma - a review. Med Sci Monit 2014; 20:103–9.

31. Meis-Kindblom JM, Kindblom LG. Angiosarcoma of soft tissue: a study of 80 cases. Am J Surg Pathol 1998;22(6):683–97.

32. Linfeng Q, Xingjie X, Henry D, et al. Cardiac angiosarcoma: A case report and review of current treatment. Medicine (Baltimore) 2019;98(49):e18193.

33. Araoz PA, Eklund HE, Welch TJ, et al. CT and MR imaging of primary cardiac malignancies. Radiographics 1999;19(6):1421–34.

34. Yu JF, Cui H, Ji GM, et al. Clinical and imaging manifestations of primary cardiac angiosarcoma. BMC Med Imaging 2019;19(1):16.

35. Zhang R, Li L, Li X, et al. Primary cardiac angiosarcoma: A case report. Medicine (Baltimore) 2017; 96(42):e7352.

36. Kumar P, Singh A, Deshmukh A, et al. Cardiac MRI for the evaluation of cardiac neoplasms. Clin Radiol 2020;75(4):241–53.

37. Antonuzzo L, Rotella V, Mazzoni F, et al. Primary cardiac angiosarcoma: a fatal disease. Case Rep Med 2009;2009:591512.

38. Blackmon SH, Reardon MJ. Surgical treatment of primary cardiac sarcomas. Tex Heart Inst J 2009; 36(5):451–2.

39. Kollar A, Jones RL, Stacchiotti S, et al. Pazopanib in advanced vascular sarcomas: an EORTC Soft Tissue and Bone Sarcoma Group (STBSG) retrospective analysis. Acta Oncol 2017;56(1):88–92.

40. Grebenc ML, Rosado de Christenson ML, Burke AP, et al. Primary cardiac and pericardial neoplasms: radiologic-pathologic correlation. Radiographics 2000;20(4):1073–103 [quiz: 1110-1, 1112].

41. Okamoto K, Kato S, Katsuki S, et al. Malignant fibrous histiocytoma of the heart: case report and review of 46 cases in the literature. Intern Med 2001; 40(12):1222–6.

42. Simpson L, Kumar SK, Okuno SH, et al. Malignant primary cardiac tumors: review of a single institution experience. Cancer 2008;112(11):2440–6.

43. Bakaeen FG, Jaroszewski DE, Rice DC, et al. Outcomes after surgical resection of cardiac sarcoma in the multimodality treatment era. J Thorac Cardiovasc Surg 2009;137(6):1454–60.

44. Jeudy J, Burke AP, Frazier AA. Cardiac Lymphoma. Radiol Clin North Am 2016;54(4):689–710.

45. Ikeda H, Nakamura S, Nishimaki H, et al. Primary lymphoma of the heart: case report and literature review. Pathol Int 2004;54(3):187–95.

46. Burke A, Tavora F, Maleszewski JJ, et al. Tumors of the heart and great vessels. American Registry of Pathology; 2015. Available at: https://www.arppress.org/tumors-heart-great-vessels-p/4f22.htm.

47. Carras S, Berger F, Chalabreysse L, et al. Primary cardiac lymphoma: diagnosis, treatment and outcome in a modern series. Hematol Oncol 2017; 35(4):510–9.

48. Ceresoli GL, Ferreri AJ, Bucci E, et al. Primary cardiac lymphoma in immunocompetent patients: diagnostic and therapeutic management. Cancer 1997; 80(8):1497–506.

49. D'Souza MM, Jaimini A, Bansal A, et al. FDG-PET/CT in lymphoma. Indian J Radiol Imaging 2013;23(4): 354–65.

50. Petrich A, Cho SI, Billett H. Primary cardiac lymphoma: an analysis of presentation, treatment, and outcome patterns. Cancer 2011;117(3):581–9.

# Imaging of the Posterior/ Paravertebral Mediastinum

Brett W. Carter, MD[a],*, John P. Lichtenberger III, MD[b]

## KEYWORDS

• Mediastinum • Compartments • CT • MR imaging • PET/CT • ITMIG

## KEY POINTS

- A wide variety of neoplastic and non-neoplastic entities may originate from the paravertebral mediastinum.
- Neurogenic neoplasms are the most common paravertebral compartment masses and typically represent peripheral nerve sheath tumors, which manifest as smooth, round or oval masses in the paravertebral region on computed tomography.
- Non-neurogenic primary and secondary neoplasms are much less common than neurogenic tumors in the paravertebral mediastinum and may arise from osseous structures or soft tissues.
- Spinal infections typically are due to bacterial infections and result in ill-defined soft tissue, unorganized fluid, and/or loculated collections.
- Intrathoracic meningoceles are associated with neurofibromatosis type 1 and manifest as a unilocular mass of fluid attenuation, often associated with vertebral anomalies, such as hemivertebrae, butterfly vertebra, or spina bifida.

## INTRODUCTION

The paravertebral mediastinal compartment contains several vascular and nonvascular organs and anatomic structures from which a wide variety of anatomic variants and abnormalities may arise. It has been well established that a combination of lesion localization, characterization with cross-sectional imaging modalities, and correlation with demographics and other clinical information typically enable the development of a focused differential diagnosis. The first step in this process is identifying the compartment from which a mediastinal mass originates, which can be accomplished by employing the mediastinal compartment classification scheme created by the International Thymic Malignancy Interest Group (ITMIG), which has been accepted as a standard.[1]

The following boundaries have been defined for the paravertebral mediastinal compartment[1]: superiorly, the thoracic inlet[2]; inferiorly, the diaphragm[3]; anteriorly, the posterior boundaries of the visceral compartment; and[4] posterolaterally, a vertical line along the posterior margin of the chest wall at the lateral aspect of the transverse processes. With these anatomic landmarks in mind, the most significant organs and anatomic structures contained in the paravertebral compartment include the thoracic spine and paravertebral soft tissues. The most common masses and other abnormalities originating from the paravertebral compartment are neurogenic neoplasms, non-neurogenic tumors, infections (discitis/osteomyelitis), and those related to trauma (hematoma), although a wide variety of miscellaneous lesions related to other underlying conditions (such as extramedullary hematopoiesis) are possible.

[a] Department of Thoracic Imaging, MD Anderson Cancer Center, 1515 Holcombe Boulevard, Unit 1478, Houston, TX 77030, USA; [b] Department of Radiology, The George Washington University Hospital, 900 23rd Street Northwest, Suite G 2092, Washington, DC 20037, USA
* Corresponding author. 1515 Holcombe Boulevard, Unit 1478, Houston, TX 77030.
E-mail address: bcarter2@mdanderson.org

Radiol Clin N Am 59 (2021) 243–249
https://doi.org/10.1016/j.rcl.2020.11.010
0033-8389/21/© 2020 Elsevier Inc. All rights reserved.

## IMAGING OF PARAVERTEBRAL ABNORMALITIES
### General Considerations

Lesions in the paravertebral mediastinum typically originate from the thoracic spine and paravertebral soft tissues, the most common of which are neurogenic neoplasms. Primary lymphoma and bone tumors as well as metastatic disease are less common but may be seen. Non-neoplastic abnormalities include etiologies such as infections of the spine of the spine; cystic lesions, such as intrathoracic meningocele and neurenteric cyst; and extramedullary hematopoiesis. Although the composition, morphology, and other imaging features may be sufficient to make a specific diagnosis, in other cases, correlation with clinical information is necessary.

### Neurogenic Neoplasms

Neurogenic neoplasms are the most common paravertebral compartment masses and represent 20% and 35% of all adult and pediatric mediastinal neoplasms, respectively.[2] Most of these lesions (70%–80%) are benign. Peripheral nerve sheath tumors originate from spinal or proximal intercostal nerves, less commonly from the vagus, recurrent laryngeal, or phrenic nerves, and represent 70% of mediastinal neurogenic neoplasms.[2] Multiple neurofibromas may be encountered in patients with neurofibromatosis type 1. On computed tomography (CT), peripheral nerve sheath neoplasms, such as neurofibroma or schwannomas, manifest as smooth, round or oval masses in the paravertebral region that may exhibit a dumbbell shape and communicate with the spinal canal (**Fig. 1**). Cystic changes or hemorrhage may result in regions of internal heterogeneity and are more common in schwannomas than in neurofibromas.[2] Although pressure erosion of adjacent ribs or vertebrae and enlargement of the neural foramina may be seen, these are benign findings and should be differentiated from bone invasion and destruction, which are typical of malignancies. MR imaging offers the advantage of showing the extent of intraspinal/extradural extension and may be used in some instances to distinguish between the types of peripheral nerve sheath tumors based on unique signs (**Figs. 2 and 3**). For example, multiple small, ringlike structures of low signal intensity representing fascicular bundles is known as the *fascicular sign* and typically is seen with schwannomas. On the other hand, the combination of central low signal intensity and surrounding peripheral high signal intensity is termed the *target sign,* and is seen more commonly with neurofibromas than with schwannomas.

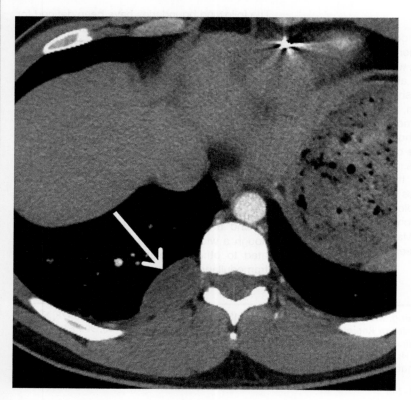

**Fig.        1. Neurofibroma.** Contrast-enhanced axial CT of the chest of a 43-year-old man demonstrates an elongate low-attenuation mass in the right paravertebral mediastinum (*arrow*). Biopsy revealed neurofibroma, a benign peripheral nerve sheath tumor that is one of the most common paravertebral masses.

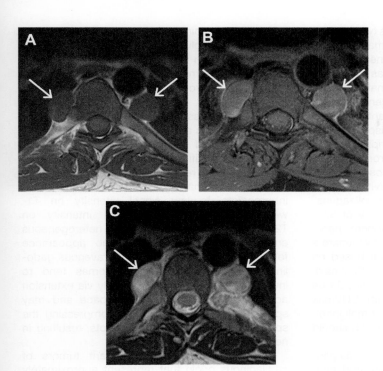

**Fig. 2.** Neurofibromas in neurofibromatosis type 1. (*A*) Axial T1-weighted, (*B*) postcontrast T1-weighted, and (*C*) T2-weighted MR images of a patient with neurofibromatosis type 1 demonstrate multiple paravertebral neurofibromas (*arrows*) that enhance and show predominantly high T2 signal intensity although internal regions of low T2 signal also are present.

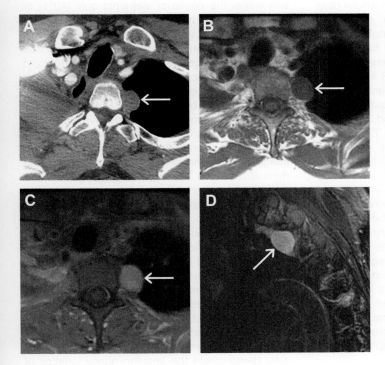

**Fig. 3.** Schwannoma. (*A*) Contrast-enhanced axial CT of the chest of a 56-year-old woman with a history of lung cancer shows a well-circumscribed low-attenuation lesion in the left paravertebral mediastinum (*arrow*). Axial T1-weighted (*B*) and postcontrast T1-weighted MR images (*C*) and sagittal T2-weighted MR image (*D*) demonstrate homogeneous enhancement and high T2 signal intensity (*arrows*). Biopsy revealed schwannoma.

For patients with neurofibromatosis type 1, there is a 10% lifetime risk of developing a malignant peripheral nerve sheath tumor. If a neurofibroma demonstrates imaging findings such as sudden increase in size, development of internal heterogeneity, and/or invasion of adjacent tissues, malignant transformation to a malignant peripheral nerve sheath neoplasm should be suspected. Differentiation between a malignant peripheral nerve sheath tumor and a benign neurofibroma may be accomplished with fluorodeoxyglucose PET/CT, with 1 study demonstrating sensitivity of 95% and specificity of 72%.[3] Warbey and colleagues[4] found sensitivity of 97% and specificity of 87% for the detection of malignant peripheral nerve sheath neoplasms. Additionally, the investigators suggested the following management based on maximum standardized uptake value (SUVmax): (1) lesions with SUVmax less than 2.5 should be considered benign; (2) masses with SUVmax greater than 3.5 should be considered malignant; and (3) lesions with SUVmax of 2.5 to 3.5 should undergo surveillance imaging.[4]

Sympathetic ganglion neoplasms, such as ganglioneuromas, ganglioneuroblastomas, and neuroblastomas, and neuroendocrine neoplasms, such as paragangliomas, are other neurogenic tumors that may arise in the paravertebral mediastinum; however, these are much less common than peripheral nerve sheath tumors and many of the imaging features of these tumors are nonspecific, necessitating histologic assessment for diagnosis. Paragangliomas arise from clusters of neuroendocrine cells called paraganglia and are classified by location and secretory function. On contrast-enhanced CT, paragangliomas demonstrate intense enhancement. On MR imaging, lesions exhibit a salt-and-pepper appearance from enhancing tumor and signal flow voids of blood vessels on T1-weighted imaging and high signal intensity (light bulb appearance) on T2-weighted imaging.[5]

## Other Neoplasms

Non-neurogenic primary and secondary neoplasms also may be encountered in the paravertebral mediastinal compartment but are much less common than neurogenic tumors. The most common primary tumors to occur in this region may be classified as either osseous or soft tissue in origin, with chordoma and chondrosarcoma included in the former and lymphoma in the latter.

Although chordomas of the vertebral bodies are rare, they are the second most common primary malignancy in the spine following lymphoproliferative neoplasms.[6]

The thoracic spine is the most infrequent portion of the spine involved, following the cervical and lumbar spine. On CT, chordomas typically manifest as well circumscribed destructive lytic lesions that may be heterogeneous due to the presence of necrosis and/or hemorrhage. The associated expansile soft tissue mass is often much larger than the osseous abnormality.

Internal foci of high attenuation appearing as intratumoral calcifications may be present, which are thought to represent sequestra of normal bone. On MR imaging, chordomas demonstrate intermediate to low signal intensity on T1-weighted imaging, high signal intensity on T2-weighted imaging, and heterogeneous enhancement with a honeycomb appearance following the administration of intravenous gadolinium contrast material. Chordomas tend to involve more than 1 vertebral body via extension across the intervertebral disc space and may spread to the epidural space, compressing the spinal cord or along the nerve roots, resulting in neural foraminal expansion.

Chondrosarcomas are malignant tumors of cartilaginous origin that represent approximately 25% of all primary malignant neoplasms of bone, although involvement of the spine accounts for only approximately 7% of cases.[7] The thoracic spine is the most frequent portion of the spine affected. The posterior elements and vertebral body are involved in 45% of cases whereas location within the posterior elements only (40%) or the vertebral body only (15%) is less common. On CT, tumors are lytic approximately 50% of the time and contain internal calcifications that may be in a rings and arcs pattern or popcorn morphology. Endosteal scalloping may be present and affects greater than two-thirds of the cortical thickness of the bone affected. Higher-grade tumors may demonstrate a permeative pattern of bone destruction. On MR imaging, lesions demonstrate low to intermediate signal on T1-weighted imaging, high signal intensity in the regions without mineralization on T2-weighted imaging, and heterogeneous enhancement following the administration of intravenous gadolinium contrast material.

Non-neurogenic soft tissue tumors affecting the paravertebral mediastinum are uncommon and tend to represent lymphoma, metastatic disease, or a variety of unusual neoplasms. When lymphoma arises from the mediastinum as a primary malignant neoplasm, the paravertebral compartment is the least common site of involvement (**Fig. 4**). A wide variety of neoplasms may metastasize to the paravertebral mediastinum and typically demonstrate the imaging characteristics of

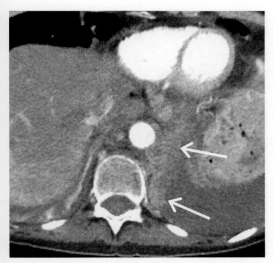

**Fig. 4.** Lymphoma. Contrast-enhanced axial CT of the chest of a 62-year-old man with a remote history of primary mediastinal (thymic) lymphoma demonstrates extensive lobular soft tissue in the left paravertebral mediastinum (*arrows*) representing recurrent disease and spread to the other mediastinal compartments.

the primary tumor and metastases elsewhere in the body (**Fig. 5**).

## Spinal Infections

Infections of the bone and/or soft tissues of the spine usually result from bacterial organisms

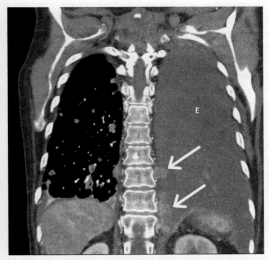

**Fig. 5.** Metastatic disease. Contrast-enhanced coronal CT of the chest of a 54-year-old man with metastatic renal cell carcinoma demonstrates numerous enhancing metastases in the left paravertebral mediastinum (*arrows*). Note the large left pleural effusion (E) and other bilateral metastases.

and are seen in patients with 1 or more risk factors, such as diabetes, autoimmune diseases, malignancy, immunosuppression, and intravenous drug use.[8] Tuberculosis should be considered in the setting of immunodeficiency, in particular, human immunodeficiency virus (HIV) infection. It is estimated that 60% of HIV-positive patients with tuberculosis have skeletal involvement, with the most commonly involved site the spine (in approximately 50% of cases).

On cross-sectional imaging, the most common abnormalities reported in spinal infections include ill-defined soft tissue, unorganized fluid, and/or loculated collections. One or more of these imaging findings typically are seen in combination with clinical symptoms such as back pain, fever, and malaise. On CT, early and late findings of spinal infection have been described, with soft tissue infiltration of the paravertebral fat and intervertebral disc hypoattenuation present in the former, and osseous erosion, disc space narrowing, and sequestrum formation seen in the latter.[8] In the setting of involvement of the posterior elements, a large soft tissue mass located in the prevertebral and paravertebral regions that is out of proportion to the extent of bone destruction, and intervertebral disc space narrowing, tuberculosis should be suspected as the causative agent and can help differentiate it from pyogenic infection. Additionally, Pott disease of the spine should be considered when calcification is present but new bone formation or sclerosis is absent.[9,10]

## Intrathoracic Meningocele

An intrathoracic meningocele is formed from anomalous herniation of the leptomeninges through a defect in an intervertebral foramen or vertebral body defect.[11] These lesions are associated with neurofibromatosis type 1 and are more common in adults than children. On CT, a meningocele manifests as a unilocular mass of fluid attenuation and is associated with vertebral anomalies, such as hemivertebrae, butterfly vertebra, or spina bifida (**Fig. 6**). Although intrathoracic meningoceles may be difficult to distinguish from other low-attenuation abnormalities in the paravertebral mediastinum, such as neurenteric cysts and neurogenic neoplasms, correlation with clinical information, such as associated neurofibromatosis type 1, is helpful. When in doubt, CT, MR imaging, or myelography performed after intraspinal injection of contrast material can be used to demonstrate the presence of a meningocele.[12]

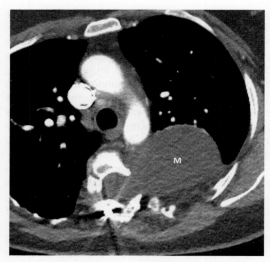

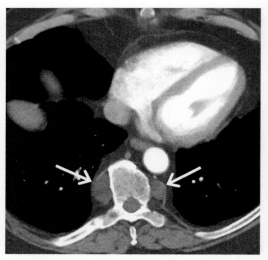

**Fig. 6.** Intrathoracic meningocele. Contrast-enhanced axial CT of the chest of a 39-year-old woman with neurofibromatosis type 1 shows a well-defined low-attenuation mass extending from the spinal canal into the left paravertebral mediastinum (M), representing an intrathoracic meningocele. Note the post-surgical changes in the spine.

**Fig. 7.** Extramedullary hematopoiesis. Contrast-enhanced axial CT of the chest of a 43-year-old man with myelofibrosis demonstrates soft tissue masses (*arrows*) in the paravertebral mediastinum bilaterally, consistent with extramedullary hematopoiesis. Note the ill-defined regions of internal low-attenuation representing fat in these long-standing lesions.

## Extramedullary Hematopoiesis

Extramedullary hematopoiesis is a process that is seen most commonly in the setting of a hematologic disorder resulting in bone marrow replacement, such as myelofibrosis or chronic myelogenous leukemia, or hemolytic anemia, including thalassemia, sickle cell anemia, and hereditary spherocytosis.[13] On CT, extramedullary hematopoiesis manifests as masses adjacent to thoracic vertebrae and/or ribs in the paravertebral mediastinum that are variable in size and number. Due to the high internal vascularity, these lesions typically enhance following the administration of intravenous iodinated contrast material. Heterogeneous attenuation and/or enhancement, however, may be encountered in the setting of iron deposition and fat infiltration in long-standing lesions[14] (**Fig. 7**). Due to the vascular nature of the lesions and the need to avoid biopsy in some cases, imaging with technetium Tc 99m sulfur colloid bone marrow scanning and single-photon emission CT/CT bone marrow scanning may be employed to confirm the presence of functioning hematopoietic tissue and confirm the diagnosis. Associated abnormalities, such as the presence of autosplenectomy in patients with sickle cell disease, are invaluable in suggesting the diagnosis.

## Other Cystic Lesions

Several uncommon disease processes may result in cystic abnormalities in the paravertebral compartment and should be considered in the appropriate clinical scenario. On CT, mediastinal abscess should be considered when a low-attenuation mass is identified in a patient who has recently undergone surgery or who has a history of esophageal perforation. Internal foci of air and/or communication with coexisting subphrenic abscesses or empyema may be present.[15] When a diagnosis remains uncertain, percutaneous needle aspiration may be necessary to exclude other etiologies, such as postoperative seroma or hematoma. Pancreatic pseudocyst should be considered when a thin-walled low-attenuation or high-attenuation mass is present and develops over a short period of time in a patient with the clinical picture of pancreatitis.[16] These lesions contain pancreatic secretions, blood, and necrotic material and may result in the regions of high attenuation. Spread occurs through the esophageal or aortic hiatus although separate intra-abdominal pseudocysts may or may not be present.

## SUMMARY

Paravertebral mediastinal masses include a wide range of benign and malignant entities, some of which may be identified incidentally on imaging examinations performed for unrelated reasons. Combining available tools, such as localizing mediastinal masses to the paravertebral compartment, characterizing them with cross-sectional imaging techniques, and correlating the imaging findings with demographics and other clinical history, typically enable the radiologist to create a focused differential diagnosis. Clinical imagers, however, must be familiar with these concepts in order to help guide subsequent imaging and/or intervention and treatment planning for neoplasms and other abnormalities.

## DISCLOSURE

Nothing to disclose for all authors.

## REFERENCES

1. Carter BW, Tomiyama N, Bhora FY, et al. A modern definition of mediastinal compartments. J Thorac Oncol 2014;9(9 suppl 2):S97–101.

2. Strollo DC, Rosado-de-Christenson ML, Jett JR. Primary mediastinal tumors. II. Tumors of the middle and posterior mediastinum. Chest 1997;112(5): 1344–57.

3. Bredella MA, Torriani M, Hornicek F, et al. Value of PET in the assessment of patients with neurofibromatosis type 1. AJR Am J Roentgenol 2007;189(4): 928–35.

4. Warbey VS, Ferner RE, Dunn JT, et al. [18F]FDG PET/CT in the diagnosis of malignant peripheral nerve sheath tumours in neurofibromatosis type-1. Eur J Nucl Med Mol Imaging 2009;36(5):751–7.

5. Sahdev A, Sohaib A, Monson JP, et al. CT and MR imaging of unusual locations of extra-adrenal paragangliomas (pheochromocytomas). Eur Radiol 2005;15(1):85–92.

6. Murphey MD, Andrews CL, Flemming DJ, et al. From the archives of the AFIP. Primary tumors of the spine: radiologic pathologic correlation. Radiographics 1996;16(5):1131–58.

7. Murphey MD, Walker EA, Wilson AJ, et al. From the archives of the AFIP: imaging of primary chondrosarcoma: radiologic-pathologic correlation. Radiographics 2003;23(5):1245–78.

8. Meyer CA, Vagal AS, Seaman D. Put your back into it: pathologic conditions of the spine at chest CT. RadioGraphics 2011;31(5):1425–41.

9. De Backer AI, Mortelé KJ, Vanschoubroeck IJ, et al. Tuberculosis of the spine: CT and MR imaging features. JBR-BTR 2005;88(2):92–7.

10. Engin G, Acunaş B, Acunaş G, et al. Imaging of extrapulmonary tuberculosis. RadioGraphics 2000; 20(2):471–88 [quiz 529–530, 532].

11. Juanpere S, Cañete N, Ortuño P, et al. A diagnostic approach to the mediastinal masses. Insights Imaging 2013;4(1):29–52.

12. Webb WR. Diseases of the mediastinum. In: Putman CE, Ravin CE, editors. Textbook of diagnostic imaging. 2nd edition. Philadelphia (PA): Saunders; 1994. p. 428–47.

13. Berkmen YM, Zalta BA. Case 126: extramedullary hematopoiesis. Radiology 2007;245(3):905–8.

14. Georgiades CS, Neyman EG, Francis IR, et al. Typical and atypical presentations of extramedullary hemopoiesis. AJR Am J Roentgenol 2002;179(5): 1239–43.

15. Glazer HS, Siegel MJ, Sagel SS. Low-attenuation mediastinal masses on CT. AJR Am J Roentgenol 1989;152(6):1173–7.

16. Kirchner SG, Heller RM, Smith CW. Pancreatic pseudocyst of the mediastinum. Radiology 1977;123(1): 37–42.

# Added Value of Magnetic Resonance Imaging for the Evaluation of Mediastinal Lesions

Allen P. Heeger, DO, Jeanne B. Ackman, MD*

## KEYWORDS

- MR imaging • Mediastinum • Mediastinal MR imaging • Mediastinal mass • Thymic hyperplasia
- Thymic cyst • Thymoma

## KEY POINTS

- Magnetic resonance (MR) imaging can add diagnostic specificity to the evaluation of indeterminate mediastinal lesions on radiography and computed tomography, serving as a means of virtual biopsy.
- Mediastinal MR imaging can assist in directing intervention and guiding surgical management, and can serve as a means of surveillance without exposure to ionizing radiation.
- Dynamic MR imaging during free breathing amplifies assessment of lesion invasiveness and phrenic nerve involvement.
- Using MR imaging to characterize mediastinal lesions noninvasively can have a significant impact on patient care.

Video content accompanies this article at http://www.radiologic.theclinics.com.

## INTRODUCTION

Imaging of the mediastinum has long relied on chest radiography (CXR) and computed tomography (CT) to triage benign, malignant, and indeterminate lesions in terms of clinical management. A thorough understanding of the anatomy and classification schemas has allowed radiologists to localize and differentiate lesions, narrowing diagnostic possibilities. However, some lesions remain indeterminate, many of which are benign. Before the use of magnetic resonance (MR) imaging, many indeterminate mediastinal lesions required longitudinal CT follow-up, exposure to repeated doses of ionizing radiation, and often unnecessary surgical excision.[1] MR imaging has the capacity to further characterize these indeterminate lesions and guide clinical management, on account of its superior soft tissue contrast and tissue characterization properties.[2]

## DISCUSSION

### Nature of the Problem: Limitations of Computed Tomography and the Added Value of Magnetic Resonance Imaging

One primary limitation of CT that must be considered is the ionizing radiation required to produce diagnostic images. Although progress has been made since the inception of CT to reduce radiation dose, diagnostic ionizing radiation exposure over a patient's lifetime remains a concern because of higher cancer risk.[3–8] Adhering to the guiding principle of radiation safety, as low as reasonably

No relevant financial disclosures.
Department of Radiology, Division of Thoracic Imaging and Intervention, Harvard Medical School, Massachusetts General Hospital, Founders House 202, 55 Fruit Street, Boston, MA 02114, USA
* Corresponding author.
E-mail address: jackman@mgh.harvard.edu

Radiol Clin N Am 59 (2021) 251–277
https://doi.org/10.1016/j.rcl.2020.11.001
0033-8389/21/© 2020 Elsevier Inc. All rights reserved.

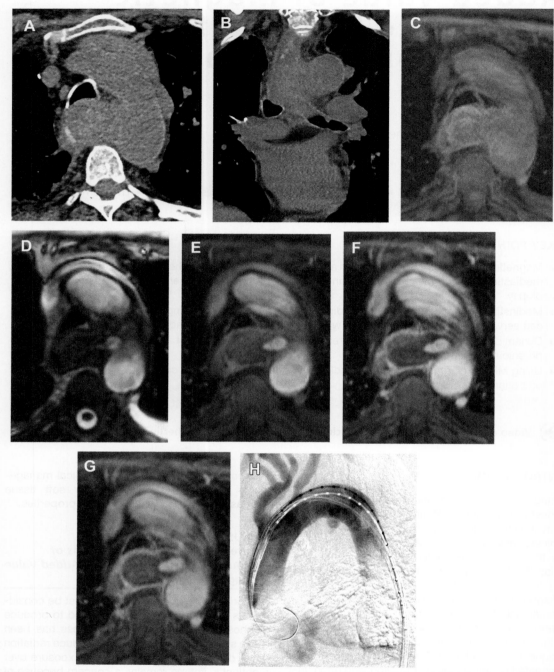

Fig. 1. Superior soft tissue contrast of MR imaging allows delineation of structures. Acute mediastinitis and aortic mycotic pseudoaneurysm diagnosed at MR imaging following indeterminate CT findings. Unenhanced axial (*A*) and coronal (*B*) CT scans of the chest of an 80-year-old man with dysphagia and septic shock reveal indeterminate, amorphous soft tissue attenuation material in the visceral mediastinum along the medial aspect of the aortic arch. Differential considerations included an esophageal malignancy and confluent mediastinal lymphadenopathy. MR imaging was pursued after stabilization of labile blood pressure and improvement of acute kidney injury 5 days later. MR imaging showed the masslike material to be (*C*) peripherally T1-hyperintense and centrally T1-isointense on precontrast fat-saturated T1-weighted images and to efface fat planes along the esophagus and the aorta. Steady state free-precession (SSFP) image (*D*) revealed a focal irregular outpouching of the medial wall of the aortic arch with intrinsic signal following that of the blood pool on this sequence and all subsequent

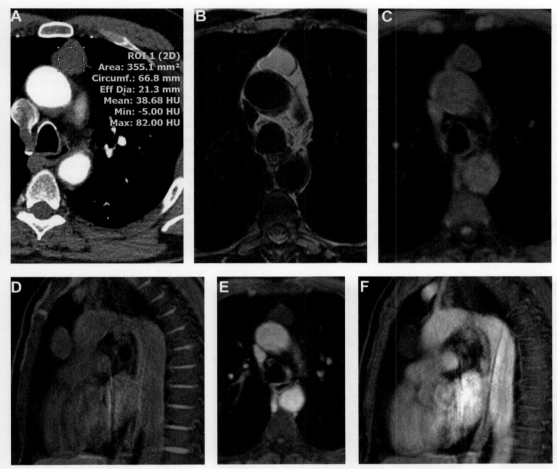

**Fig. 2.** Distinction of cystic from solid lesions. Indeterminate thymic mass on CT shown to be a unilocular protein-aceous or hemorrhagic cyst by MR imaging. Contrast-enhanced axial CT of the chest (*A*) shows a homogeneous-attenuation, 39-Hounsfield-unit (HU) mass in the central aspect of the thymic bed. Differential considerations include a thymic cyst and thymic epithelial neoplasm, with a metastasis less likely in the absence of other lymph-adenopathy in this 51-year-old woman undergoing staging for appendiceal carcinoma. Axial electrocardiogram (ECG)-gated double inversion recovery (DIR) T2-weighted (*B*), axial (*C*), and sagittal (*D*) precontrast, fat-saturated, T1-weighted MR images and corresponding postcontrast fat-saturated T1-weighted DCE MR images (*E, F*) show the mass to be of intermediate T1 signal and homogeneously T2-hyperintense, with enhancement of its smooth, thin wall and no internal enhancement, proving the mass to be a thymic bed cyst. ROI, region of interest.

achievable, continued efforts must be made to limit radiation exposure throughout each patient's lifetime. The lack of ionizing radiation use and exposure by MR imaging is therefore compelling.

Although CT is able to quickly and noninvasively provide cross-sectional evaluation of lesions, its soft tissue contrast and tissue characterization capability are inferior to those of MR imaging. As

a result, CT does not always allow confident defi-nition of a lesion's relationship to surrounding structures (**Fig. 1**), definitive placement of a lesion into a specific mediastinal compartment, and confident delineation of a lesion's borders and invasiveness, all of which can have profound diag-nostic and prognostic implications affecting clin-ical management.

---

pulse sequences. Postcontrast fat-saturated T1-weighted DCE images (*E–G*) performed at 20 seconds (*E*), 1 minute (*F*), and 5 minutes (*G*) after intravenous (IV) gadolinium administration confirmed the lesion to be an aortic pseu-doaneurysm (mycotic). The patient underwent emergent catheter angiography (*H*) and thoracic endovascular aortic repair.

Determining a lesion's internal characteristics is also imperative to diagnosis. Although CT does a good job delineating structures with starkly differing attenuation, such as air, macroscopic fat, water, and bone, it is less proficient at differentiating tissues of similar attenuation, of which there are many. A stark example is the frequent inability of CT, whether performed without or with intravenous (IV) iodinated contrast, to differentiate a hyperattenuating or isoattenuating cyst from a solid lesion, which typically occurs when the cyst contains sufficient proteinaceous or mineral material (eg, hemorrhage, calcium oxalate, manganese, magnesium) (**Fig. 2**).[9]

Use of IV iodinated contrast contributes to tissue characterization and can thereby narrow the differential diagnosis. Chest CT imaging without and with IV contrast and dynamic contrast enhancement (DCE) are seldom performed because of the consequential doubling and quadrupling of ionizing radiation exposure, respectively. The inferior soft tissue contrast of CT, compared with MR imaging, additionally limits the ability of CT to detect subtle enhancement (**Fig. 3**). Dual energy techniques have shown promise in further characterizing lesions; however, inherent limitations remain.[10–12] Dynamic contrast evaluation with automatic postprocessed subtraction enables MR imaging to provide potentially valuable information regarding a lesion's temporal enhancement pattern and cellularity, without the risk conferred by added ionizing radiation exposure.

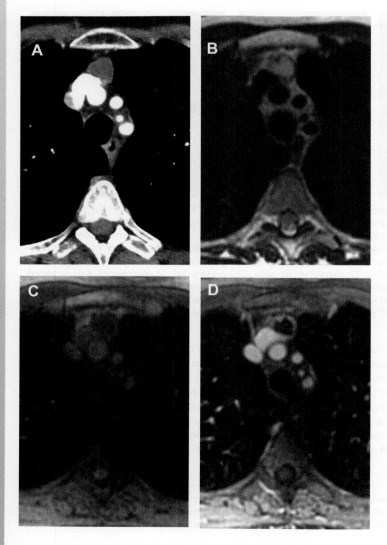

**Fig. 3.** Superior soft tissue contrast of MR imaging. Detection of nodular enhancement within a thymic cyst. Contrast-enhanced axial CT of the chest (*A*) shows a homogeneous-attenuation (53 HU) mass in the superior aspect of the thymic bed. Differential considerations include a thymic cyst and a cystic thymic epithelial neoplasm in this 58-year-old woman. Axial ECG-gated DIR T2-weighted (*B*), axial (*C*) precontrast 3D ultrafast gradient echo (GRE), fat-saturated T1-weighted and corresponding postcontrast fat-saturated T1-weighted MR images (*D*) show the mass to be T1-hypointense and homogeneously T2-hyperintense, with thin smooth wall enhancement and an eccentric area of nodular enhancement not appreciated on the CT. Excision was pursued and, despite the suspicious nodular enhancement, the lesion proved to be a benign thymic cyst.

In addition to serving as a means of noninvasive tissue sampling or virtual biopsy, preventing unnecessary diagnostic intervention, MR can facilitate diagnostic tissue sampling. Because MR imaging is proficient at identifying viable, cellular tissue, it can direct the interventionalist or surgeon to biopsy the area of highest diagnostic yield and accessibility (**Fig. 4**).[9]

Although MR imaging surpasses the ability of CT regarding lesion characterization, it has its own limitations. The greatest limiting factor is acquisition time.[13] MR imaging requires a patient to lie still for 15 to 45 minutes, which for most patients is possible; however, it limits the number of examinations that can be performed per day at a given site. Nevertheless, MR imaging pulse sequence acquisition times continue to improve with advances in software and hardware with every passing year. In addition, imaging protocols tailored to indication and accommodation of patients' needs can surmount these limitations and expedite an imaging diagnosis. In terms of tissue characterization, MR imaging's sole limitation, compared with CT, is its inability to specifically identify calcium. Because of its ability to show many other, often more important, features of a lesion, this limitation rarely has clinical implications (**Fig. 5**). Also, because MR imaging is often used to problem solve indeterminate lesions on CT, the presence or absence of calcium in a lesion is usually known.

## Imaging Protocol

Limiting the effects of cardiac and respiratory motion is essential for the acquisition of high-quality images and reduction of image-degrading artifacts (**Fig. 6**). Limiting respiratory motion artifact can be achieved via breath-hold imaging or respiratory triggering. When possible, breath-hold imaging is preferable, because it more reliably freezes respiratory motion and is a much faster image acquisition method.[9] Considerations must be made regarding coverage in order to limit breath-hold duration, because prolonged breath holds (>20 seconds) and an increased overall number of breath-hold sequences can result in patient fatigue and suboptimal image quality. Breath-hold

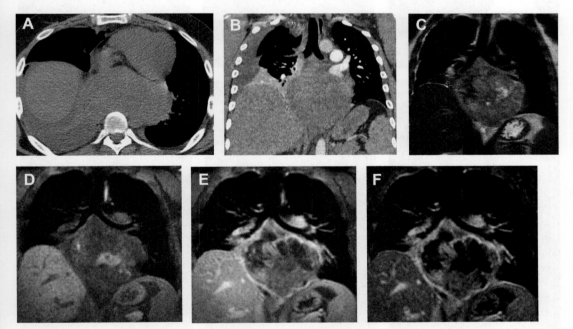

**Fig. 4.** Superior soft tissue contrast allowing identification of viable soft tissue to aid biopsy targeting. Large mediastinal sarcoma with hemorrhagic and necrotic components. Unenhanced axial (*A*) and coronal postcontrast (*B*) CT of the chest reveal a large, amorphous, heterogeneous mass in the visceral mediastinum. Coronal single-shot fast spin-echo T2-weighted (*C*), precontrast (*D*), postcontrast (*E*) fat-saturated T1-weighted 3D gradient echo, and postprocessed subtracted (*F*) MR images reveal the indeterminate mass on CT to represent a large, well-circumscribed visceral mediastinal mass with heterogeneous T1-weighted and T2-weighted signal; areas of T1-hyperintense, heterogeneous T2 signal hemorrhage; and areas of T1-hypointense, T2-hyperintense necrosis. Postcontrast subtracted images highlight the solid, cellular, enhancing components of the mass, indicating that bronchoscopic biopsy via the carina would likely be diagnostic. (*From* Ackman JB. Thoracic MRI: Technique and Approach to Diagnosis. In Shepard JAO: Thoracic Imaging, The Requisites. Philadelphia: Elsevier, p 61-87; with permission.)

imaging can be reliably achieved in most patients with preemptive coaching by the technologists and the use of supplemental, MR-compatible nasal cannula oxygen, the latter when difficulty is anticipated.[9,14]

Evaluation of mediastinal lesions by MR imaging requires complementary high-quality sequences to aid in tissue characterization. In general, these include a breath-hold two-dimensional (2D) or three-dimensional (3D) T1-weighted sequence; a breath-hold or respiratory-triggered T2-weighted sequence, with or without fat saturation; and a breath-hold pregadolinium and postgadolinium 3D ultrafast gradient echo (GRE), dynamic contrast-enhanced (DCE), fat-saturated T1-weighted sequence, with automatic postprocessed subtraction. The use of dual echo ultrafast GRE in-phase and out-of-phase chemical shift MR

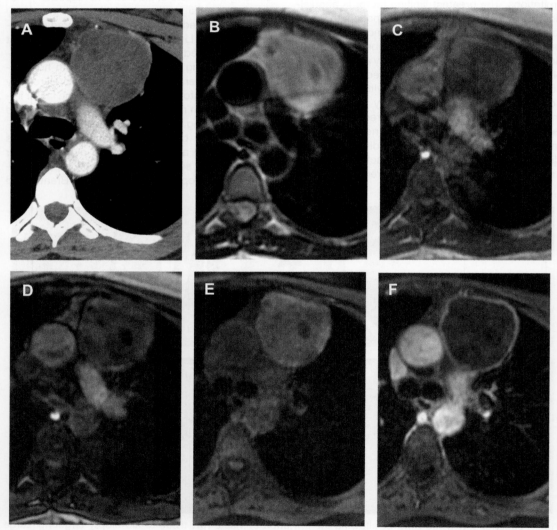

**Fig. 5.** Value of MR imaging in the characterization of fat-containing lesions. Microscopic and macroscopic fat-containing teratoma. A 42-year-old woman with an abnormal chest radiograph performed for rheumatologic evaluation. Subsequent contrast-enhanced axial CT of the chest (*A*) revealed a well-circumscribed left prevascular mediastinal lesion of mixed attenuation suggestive of solid and cystic content. ECG-gated DIR T2-weighted (*B*) MR image reveals a well-circumscribed, predominantly T2-hyperintense mass, with areas of intermediate and low signal. In-phase (*C*) and opposed-phase (*D*) T1-weighted MR images reveal suppression of signal or microscopic fat in some areas. Axial precontrast (*E*) fat-saturated T1-weighted MR image shows foci of low-signal macroscopic fat. Subsequent postcontrast images performed 5 minutes after injection (*F*) show an irregularly thickened, enhancing capsule. These features are compatible with a mature teratoma or dermoid cyst, as confirmed by subsequent surgical resection.

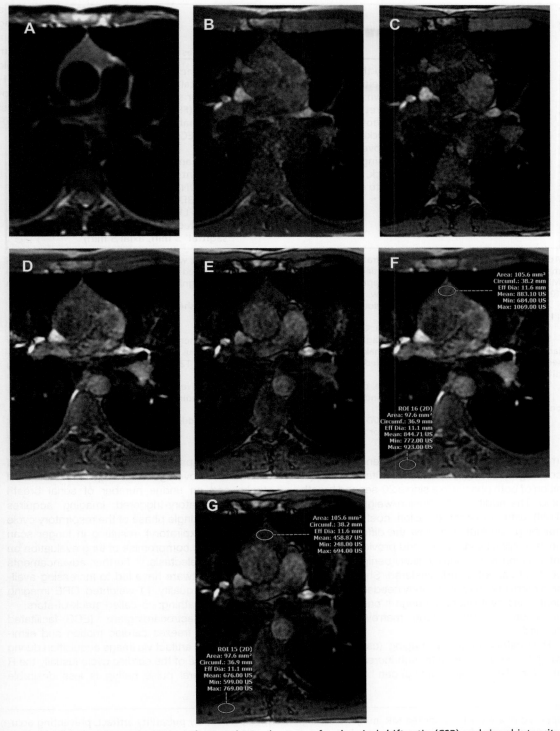

Area: 105.6 mm²
Circumf.: 38.2 mm
Eff Dia: 11.6 mm
Mean: 883.10 US
Min: 684.00 US
Max: 1069.00 US

ROI 16 (2D)
Area: 97.6 mm²
Circumf.: 36.9 mm
Eff Dia: 11.1 mm
Mean: 844.71 US
Min: 772.00 US
Max: 923.00 US

Area: 105.6 mm²
Circumf.: 38.2 mm
Eff Dia: 11.6 mm
Mean: 458.87 US
Min: 248.00 US
Max: 694.00 US

ROI 15 (2D)
Area: 97.6 mm²
Circumf.: 36.9 mm
Eff Dia: 11.1 mm
Mean: 676.00 US
Min: 599.00 US
Max: 769.00 US

**Fig. 6.** Troubleshooting pulsatility artifacts and ROI placement for chemical shift ratio (CSR) and signal intensity index (SII). Image degradation caused by pulsatility artifact. Slightly abundant thymic tissue in a 35-year-old man with left-sided ptosis and clinically suspected myasthenia gravis. A preceding CT scan showed greater-than-expected soft tissue in the thymic bed. ECG-gated DIR T2-weighted MR image (A) reveals T2-hyperintense, thymiform soft tissue in the thymic bed, with a maximum thymic lobar thickness of 1.1 cm. Initial in-phase (B) and

**Table 1**
Mediastinal magnetic resonance imaging protocol

| Protocol | Technique | Sequences |
|---|---|---|
| Mediastinum | • Coverage: solely the lesion and a few centimeters on either side, when lesion location is known; supraclavicular space down through retrocrural space (when lesion location not known)<br>• Default slice thickness: 4 mm with no overlap (2 mm overlap used for before/after T1W imaging)<br>• Interlocking neck, body, spinal matrix coils as needed to center lesion in overall coil | BH 3 plane localizer<br>BH sagittal and axial balanced gradient echo or steady state free precession (SSFP) (FIESTA/true FISP/b-FFE)[a]<br>BH coronal SSFSE/HASTE/SSTSE T2W<br>BH axial ECG-gated DIR T2W(~20 s or 1 BH/slice)[b]<br>BH axial and sagittal[c] pre-3D ultrafast gradient echo (LAVAFLEX/DIXON/mDIXON) fat-saturated T1W DCE[d,e]<br>BH post-3D ultrafast gradient echo (LAVAFLEX/DIXON/mDIXON) fat-saturated T1W: axial 20 s, axial 1 min, sagittal[c] 3 min, axial 5 min)[f] |

Additional options: breath-hold or respiratory-triggered (RTr) axial/coronal DWI, with b values of 50, 500, 800, and automated creation of ADC map. Free-breathing (and sniffing), dynamic axial balanced gradient echo (FIESTA/true FISP/b-FFE) MR sniff test to evaluate lesional and diaphragmatic mobility. Set at single, designated coronal and/or sagittal level with 10-mm slice thickness, large field of view.

*Abbreviations:* BH, breath-hold; DIR, double inversion recovery; SSFSE, single-shot fast spin echo; TSE, turbo spin echo; T1W, T1-weighted; T2W, T2-weighted.

[a] Order of MR acronyms presentation: GE/Siemens/Philips.

[b] Substitute radially acquired T2W imaging (PROPELLER/BLADE/Multivane) when full chest coverage is needed and for large masses, when extent of coverage makes ECG-gated DIR T2W imaging onerous on account of the number of serial 20-second breath-hold that would be needed to cover the lesion. Can also use this T2W sequence when a patient is having difficulty breath-holding in general.

[c] Orthogonal plane subject to change, depending on location of lesion relative to other important structures.

[d] All 4 series sent to Picture Archive and Communication System (PACS), including in-phase/out-of-phase T1W, water-only, and fat-only series.

[e] Optional BH before/after LAVAFLEX/DIXON/mDIXON T1W coronal can be added or substituted.

[f] Built-in postprocessed subtraction for all DCE series.

imaging for the T1-weighted sequence allows full coverage of most lesions and simultaneous acquisition of both phases in a single 20-second breath-hold. The addition of diffusion-weighted imaging (DWI) with apparent diffusion coefficient (ADC) mapping can further narrow the differential diagnosis in specific instances and provide reassuring information with regard to likely benignity when IV contrast cannot be administered. Short tau inversion recovery imaging is rarely needed for mediastinal mass evaluation, although it can be useful if detection of subtle bone marrow edema is needed.

Respiratory-triggered imaging (usually for T2-weighted sequences, although increasingly available for T1-weighted imaging) can be used when breath-hold capacity is limited or when the need for extended coverage would require multiple axial stacks and an undue number of serial breath holds. Respiratory-triggered imaging acquires data during a single phase of the respiratory cycle (usually end-expiratory), resulting in longer scan time and some compromise of lung evaluation on account of atelectasis.[14] Further advancements in scanner software have led to increasing availability of high-quality T1-weighted GRE imaging during free breathing: so-called stack-of-stars.

Effective electrocardiogram (ECG)-facilitated cardiac gating freezes cardiac motion and eliminates pulsation artifact via image acquisition during a specific phase of the cardiac cycle (usually the R wave). Peripheral pulse gating is less desirable

opposed-phase (*C*) T1-weighted MR images were significantly degraded by pulsatility artifact, preventing accurate assessment of signal intensity and calculation of the SII or CSR. To remedy this issue, the phase-encoding and frequency-encoding gradient directions were exchanged from the default anteroposterior phase-encoding direction and transverse, frequency-encoding direction. The result of this modification did not eliminate the pulsatility artifact but instead oriented it transversely (*D*, *E*) so that it no longer overlay the thymus and allowed accurate assessment of SII and CSR. Proper placement of ROIs over the thymic tissue and paraspinal musculature is shown (*F*, *G*), with careful avoidance of India ink artifact on the opposed-phase image. CSR = 0.6, SII = 48%.

because the time delay between the heartbeat and the peripheral pulse leads to less precise cardiac gating and residual pulsation artifact. Cardiac gating may be preferable for T2-weighted imaging when the field of coverage requires fewer than 10 to 14 slices, because it yields higher-quality images than respiratory-triggered, radially acquired, fast spin-echo T2-weighted images and breath-hold single-shot fast spin-echo images. This benefit comes at the cost of 1 breath-hold per slice, as opposed to no breath holding or a single breath-hold for the entire acquisition.[15]

Use of 3D ultrafast GRE, fat-saturated T1-weighted imaging allows the evaluation of dynamic contrast enhancement (DCE). These scans are acquired at selected intervals to allow evaluation of temporal enhancement characteristics. Suggested intervals include 20 seconds (angiographic phase), 1 minute, 3 minutes, and 5 minutes after injection, with automatic, postprocessed subtraction. Planes of image acquisition should be tailored to the patient-specific imaging question and usually include at least 1 orthogonal plane.

DWI can complement the aforementioned imaging sequences to further define a lesion's characteristics. Measuring signal decay related to motion of water molecules relies on gradient pulses of different intervals and intensity denoted as b values. The more b values used, the more accurate the ADC map; however, this comes at the cost of time to acquire each individual b value. A minimum of 3 b values is a reasonable

compromise. Low b values (<50) result in nearly pure perfusion-weighted imaging because of microvascular blood flow and resultant T2 shine-through.[16] The higher the b value, the more accurate the reflection of true diffusion. However, this comes at the cost of increased image noise with values greater than or equal to 1000. Thus, a range of b values greater than 0, evenly spaced less than 1000, can facilitate an accurate ADC map in the chest. Suggested b values are 50, 400, 800.

A standard mediastinal MR protocol and a thymus MR protocol, along with optional, supplementary sequences, are provided in **Tables 1** and **2**.

## Evaluation: Tissue Characterization by Magnetic Resonance Imaging

### Fat content
Mediastinal lesions are often surrounded by fat and, in some cases, contain macroscopic or microscopic fat. The use of appropriate fat suppression techniques can reduce the signal of both macroscopic and gross fat, including that present in the prevascular space and subcutaneous fat of the chest wall, and microscopic or intra-voxel fat (when fat-containing and water-containing molecules are present in the same voxel). The former is achieved by standard fat saturation and the latter is achieved by opposed-phase chemical shift MR imaging. Fat saturation highlights a lesion's signal characteristics by eliminating the competing high T1/T2 signal of the

**Table 2**
**Thymus MR imaging protocol**

| Protocol | Technique | Sequences |
|---|---|---|
| Thymus | • Coverage: limited coverage of lesion only<br>• Default slice thickness: 4 mm with no overlap (2 mm overlap used for before/after T1W DCE imaging)<br>• Interlocking neck, body, spinal matrix coils as needed to center lesion in overall coil<br>• Contrast can occasionally be avoided for follow-up of previously characterized lesions, if examination is monitored and no concerning interval change is detected on precontrast images | BH 3-plane localizer<br>BH axial balanced gradient echo (FIESTA/ true FISP/b-FFE)<br>BH coronal SSFSE/HASTE/SS TSE T2WI<br>BH axial ECG-gated double IR T2WI (~ 20 s or 1 BH/slice)[a]<br>BH axial and sagittal[b] pre-3D ultrafast gradient echo (LAVAFLEX/DIXON/ mDIXON) fat-saturated T1W[c,d]<br>BH post-3D ultrafast gradient echo (LAVAFLEX/DIXON/mDIXON) fat-saturated T1W DCE: axial 20s, axial 1 min, sagittal[b] 3 min, axial 5 min)[e] |

[a] Substitute radially acquired T2W imaging (T2WI) (PROPELLER/BLADE/MULTIVANE) for large masses, when extent of coverage makes ECG-gated DIR T2W imaging onerous on account of the number of serial 20-second breath holds that would be needed to cover the lesion. Can also use this T2W sequence when a patient is having difficulty breath-holding in general.
[b] Orthogonal plane subject to change, depending on location of lesion relative to other important structures.
[c] All 4 series sent to PACS, including in-phase/out-of-phase T1W, water-only, and fat-only series.
[d] Optional BH before/after-LAVAFLEX/DIXON/mDIXON fat-saturated T1W coronal can be added or substituted.
[e] Built-in postprocessed subtraction for all DCE sequences.

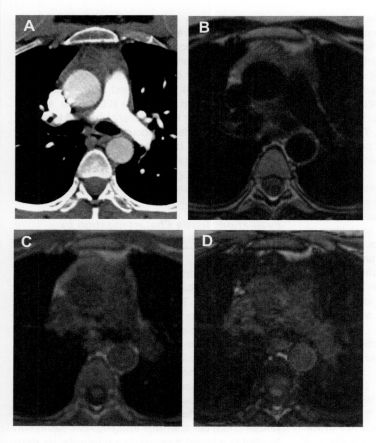

**Fig. 7.** Utility of in-phase and opposed-phase images for detection of microscopic fat (coexistent fat-containing and water-containing soft tissue in the same voxel). Rebound thymic hyperplasia in a 37-year-old woman with breast cancer and abnormally increasing thymic soft tissue on contrast-enhanced axial CT of the chest (A) more than 12 months after completion of adjuvant chemotherapy. ECG-gated DIR T2-weighted MR image (B) shows expected T2-hyperintensity relative to muscle, without underlying cyst or mass. In-phase (C) and opposed-phase (D) T1-weighted MR images reveal complete, qualitative suppression of the fatty, hyperplastic thymic tissue with signal dropout (SII) of 81%.

adjacent macroscopic fat. Identification of macroscopic or microscopic fat within a lesion often adds diagnostic specificity (see **Fig. 5**; **Fig. 7**).

Although CT can identify macroscopic fat, it cannot identify the presence of microscopic fat. As a result, it can be difficult to differentiate thymic hyperplasia from thymic tumors and lymphoma by CT, with the risk of misinterpretation of these lesions and unnecessary thymectomy.[1] Identification of microscopic fat within the thymic soft tissue in question excludes neoplasm. Consideration of the patient's age and sex must be made, when evaluating the thymus, because there is a sex difference in thymic appearance[17] and there is variation in the timeline of fatty involution of normal thymus and muscular fatty atrophy.[18]

Chemical shift MR imaging highlights the presence of microscopic fat by exploiting signal characteristics of intravoxel fat and water at different echo times using in-phase and out-of-phase GRE sequences. Initially used in evaluation of adrenal adenomas, it has more recently been recognized to be paramount for evaluation of the thymus because of thymic fatty involution with age.[17,19] Calculation of the chemical shift ratio (CSR) or

signal intensity index (SII) can be performed to differentiate normal thymus from thymic hyperplasia and thymic tumors.[20,21] This process has been further validated and refined using dual echo single-acquisition ultrafast GRE T1-weighted imaging.[22]

CSR is calculated as follows:

$$CSR = (tSI_{op}/mSI_{op})/(tSI_{in}/mSI_{in})$$

where $tSI_{op}$ is thymic signal intensity, opposed-phase; $mSI_{op}$ is muscle signal intensity, opposed-phase; $tSI_{op}$ is thymic signal intensity, in phase; and $mSI_{op}$ is muscle signal intensity, in-phase.

Based on a prospective analysis by Inaoka and colleagues,[20] CSR values less than or equal to 0.7 indicate normal or hyperplastic thymus. Values greater than 1.0 are more apt to indicate thymic neoplasms and lymphoma; however, this is not always the case. Nonsuppressing thymic hyperplasia exists not only as expected in children (whose thymuses have not yet begun to atrophy) but also in adults.[23–26] CSRs of 0.8 and 0.9 are likely benign but indeterminate and require DWI with ADC mapping to make the distinction between benignity and malignancy or serial follow-up MR imaging to confirm involution of the thymus over time. In scenarios in which normal thymus has insufficient intravoxel fat to show signal suppression on in-phase/opposed-phase imaging, the absence of restricted diffusion amidst noncystic thymic tissue virtually excludes thymic neoplasms and lymphoma[24] (Fig. 8).

The CSR calculation can be prone to error because it incorporates the signal characteristics of paraspinal musculature and is therefore affected by content of microscopic and macroscopic fat within the sampled muscle, which increases with age and/or muscle atrophy. The SII calculation does not rely on the signal intensity of paraspinal musculature and is therefore less prone to error; however, it can only be used if the chemical shift MR imaging is acquired in a single breath-hold with dual echo technique. The SII is calculated as:

$$SII = \{(tSI_{in} - tSI_{op})/tSI_{in}\} \times 100\%$$

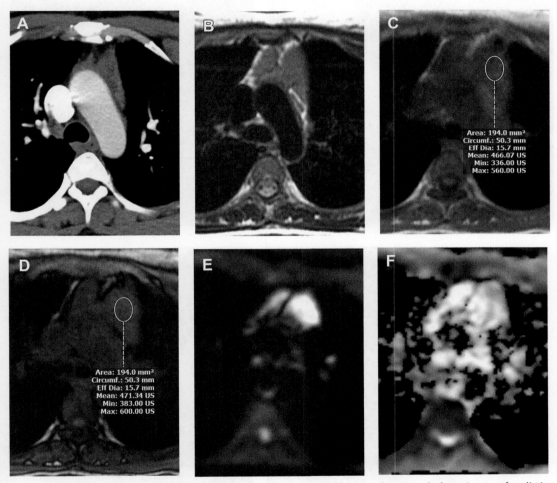

**Fig. 8.** Supplemental diagnostic value of DWI and ADC map to in-phase and opposed-phase images for distinction of thymic hyperplasia from thymic tumor. Absence of restricted diffusion in nonsuppressing thymic hyperplasia in a 40 year-old woman with history of Graves disease. Contrast-enhanced axial CT of the chest (*A*) performed for shortness of breath reveals greater-than-expected thymic tissue throughout the thymic bed, measuring 2.9 cm in maximum thymic lobar thickness. ECG-gated DIR T2-weighted MR image (*B*) reveals mildly and homogeneously T2-hyperintense tissue, without underlying cyst or mass. In-phase (*C*) and opposed-phase (*D*) GRE T1-weighted MR images with ROIs reveal no signal suppression with a calculated SII of −1%. This finding prompted further investigation with DWI because lymphoma remained a diagnostic concern. DWI (*E*) and a complementary ADC map (*F*) revealed no evidence of restricted diffusion of water molecules, virtually excluding thymic neoplasm and lymphoma. Continued monitoring after appropriate therapy showed involution of this hyperplastic thymic tissue over the next 12 months.

where $tSI_{in}$ is thymic signal intensity, in phase, and $tSI_{op}$ is thymic signal intensity, opposed phase.

Priola and colleagues[22] were able to differentiate thymic hyperplasia from tumor with 100% sensitivity and specificity using an SII value cutoff of 8.92%, with benignity indicated above this level. Greater than 10% signal suppression is a rough guide to use for confirmation of the presence of microscopic or intravoxel fat.

Essential to calculating both CSR and SII is careful placement of regions of interest (ROIs). Incorrect placement of ROI can introduce artifact and yield inaccurate results.[27] The ROI should first be placed on the out-of-phase image to avoid inclusion of chemical shift (India ink) artifact at macroscopic fat-water interfaces. Subsequently, an ROI of the same size and shape is placed within the same part of the lesion on the in-phase image.

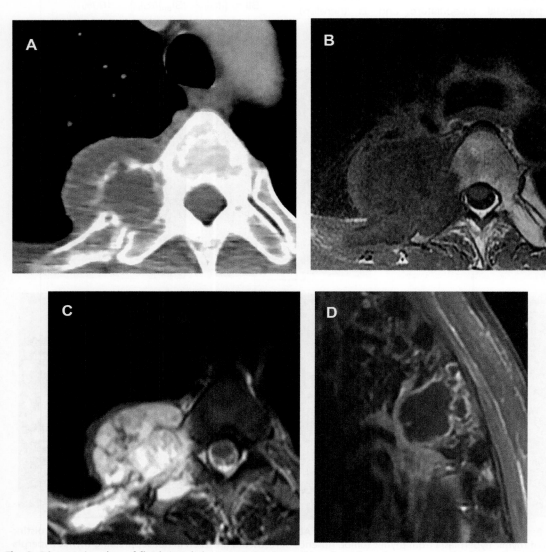

**Fig. 9.** Diagnostic value of fluid signal characteristics. Detection of cartilage in a paravertebral chondrosarcoma. Contrast-enhanced axial CT of the chest (*A*) reveals an expansile lytic lesion with cortical destruction arising from the right costovertebral joint of T4. Axial T1-weighted (*B*) and T2-weighted (*C*) MR images of this lesion reveal it to be composed of T1-hypointense, T2-hyperintense locules surrounded by T1-isointense, T2-hyperintense septae characteristic of a cartilaginous lesion. Abnormal T1-hypointense, T2-hyperintense signal involves the marrow of the adjacent rib, transverse process, and vertebral body. Sagittal fat-saturated, postcontrast, T1-weighted (*D*) MR image reveals peripheral and septal enhancement of this lesion. The tissue characteristics and extent of the lesion are not readily appreciable by the accompanying CT. (*From* Guo LQ, Ackman JB. The Pleura, Diaphragm, and Chest Wall. In Shepard JAO: Thoracic Imaging, The Requisites. Philadelphia: Elsevier, p 159-192; with permission.)

A range of CSRs and SIIs is often found in normal thymus and thymic hyperplasia, because thymic involution can be temporally and spatially heterogeneous.

### Fluid content: water, hemorrhage, proteinaceous fluid, cartilage

CT is readily able to identify fluid-containing lesions of water attenuation. However, when the fluid contains sufficient proteinaceous or mineral material, it is unable to reliably differentiate cystic from solid lesions. MR imaging allows further characterization of fluid content based on signal characteristics and can prevent unnecessary biopsy or resection of a benign entity (refer to **Fig. 2**).[1,9] In addition, the presence of epithelial or fibrous septations within a cystic lesion can be missed on CT on account of its lower soft tissue contrast. On MR imaging, serous fluid–

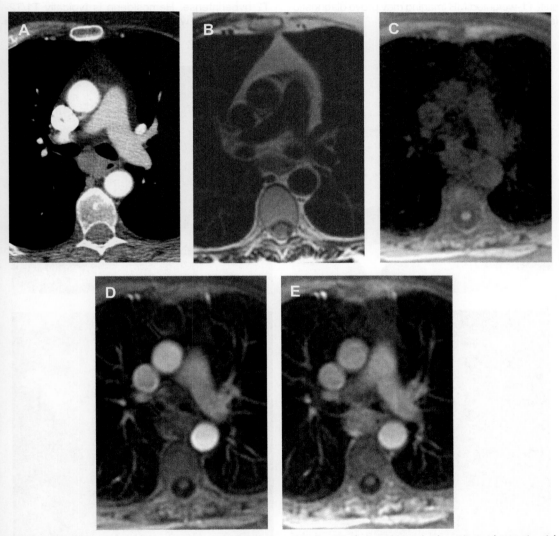

**Fig. 10.** Diagnostic value of T2-hypointense signal. Low T2 signal of densely packed, actin and myosin–rich smooth muscle fibers of an esophageal leiomyoma. Contrast-enhanced axial CT of the chest (A) of a woman with history of breast cancer reveals a rounded mass with indeterminate soft tissue attenuation in the visceral mediastinum. ECG-gated DIR T2-weighted MR image (B) shows T2-hypointense soft tissue intimately associated with the right lateral wall of the esophagus. Precontrast (C) and postcontrast fat-saturated T1-weighted MR images acquired at 20 seconds, 1 minute, 3 minutes, and 5 minutes and shown at 20 seconds (D) and 5 minutes (E) after IV gadolinium administration reveal the mass to be isointense to muscle, with mild gradual enhancement. Signal characteristics and relationship with the esophagus suggest an esophageal leiomyoma, later confirmed by endoscopy-guided needle biopsy. (*From* Guo LQ, Ackman JB. The Mediastinum. In Shepard JAO: Thoracic Imaging, The Requisites. Philadelphia: Elsevier, p 97-136; with permission.)

containing lesions are T1-hypointense and T2-hyper-intense to muscle (isointense to cerebrospinal fluid). Similarly, cartilage shows the signal characteristics of serous fluid or water (**Fig. 9**). Fat-containing fluid within dermoid cysts/mature cystic teratomas and thoracic duct cysts may approach water attenuation on CT and therefore not be distinguishable from necrotic lesions; however, by MR imaging, the frequent suppression or reduction in signal of this fluid in these lesions on opposed-phase chemical shift T1-weighted MR imaging may prove diagnostic (see **Fig. 5**).

The signal characteristics of hemorrhage depend on the acuity of the blood products and oxygenation state of the hemoglobin.[28] The high protein content of blood products in part accounts for the signal characteristics. To that effect, non-hemorrhagic proteinaceous material can also result in predictable T1-hyperintense signal characteristics. Hemorrhagic and proteinaceous material is typically T1-isointense or -hyperintense to muscle and of variable T2 signal, although usually T2-hyperintense. Hemosiderin is typically T1/T2-hypointense, which can be helpful in the

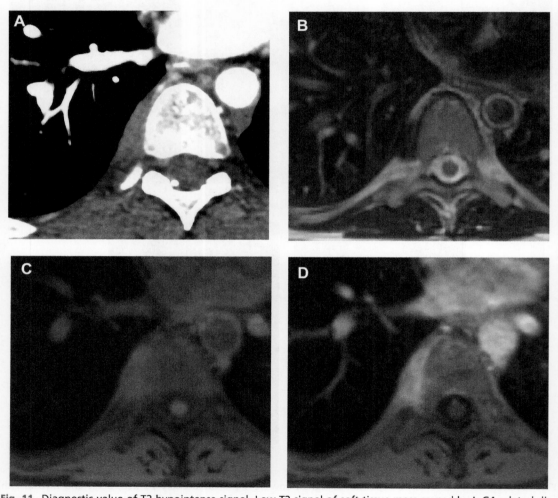

**Fig. 11.** Diagnostic value of T2-hypointense signal. Low T2 signal of soft tissue mass caused by IgG4-related disease (IgG4-RD). Contrast-enhanced axial CT of the chest (*A*) of a 55-year-old woman with autoimmune pancreatitis and multiple pulmonary nodules found to have indeterminate, abnormal, isoattenuating soft tissue in the right paravertebral mediastinum that was subsequently shown to be hypermetabolic on fluorodeoxyglucose PET/CT. Respiratory-triggered, radially acquired, axial T2-weighted fast spin-echo MR image (*B*) shows marked T2 hypointensity of the paravertebral lesion. Axial precontrast (*C*) fat-saturated T1-weighted MR image shows T1 isointensity of the lesion. Dynamic post-contrast, fat-saturated, T1-weighted MR imaging revealed gradual enhancement, peaking at 5 minutes (*D*) after injection. MR imaging findings are typical of a fibroinflammatory lesion and compatible with IgG4-RD. Subsequent CT-guided percutaneous biopsy confirmed the diagnosis.

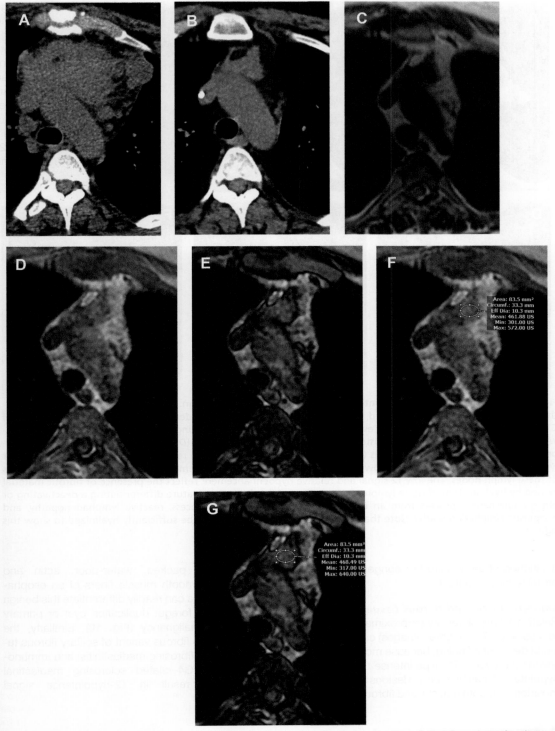

**Fig. 12.** Diagnostic value of T2 hypointensity and in-phase/opposed-phase chemical shift MR imaging for distinction of treated lymphoma from recurrent lymphoma and thymic hyperplasia. T2-hypointense signal of treated lymphoma in contradistinction to the anticipated T2 hyperintensity of lymphadenopathy present in active disease. Unenhanced axial CT of the chest of a 28-year-old woman with nodular sclerosing Hodgkin lymphoma before (*A*) and following (*B*) 6 cycles of chemotherapy reveals significant interval decrease in size of

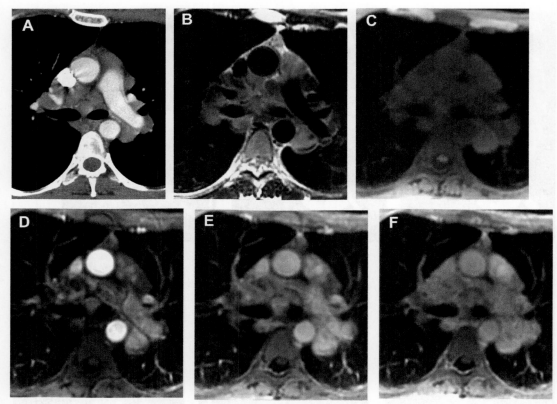

**Fig. 13.** Diagnostic value of T2 hypointensity and the dark lymph node sign: Sarcoidosis-related lymphadenopathy. Indeterminate, bulky, noncalcified, isoattenuating mediastinal lymphadenopathy on contrast-enhanced axial CT of the chest (*A*) prompted further evaluation by MR imaging in this young female patient. ECG-gated DIR T2-weighted (*B*), precontrast (*C*), and postcontrast fat-saturated T1-weighted (*D–F*) MR images performed at 20 seconds (*D*), 1 minute (*E*), and 5 minutes (*F*) after gadolinium administration reveal mediastinal and bilateral hilar lymphadenopathy, showing patchy low T2 signal and relative hypoenhancement or nonenhancement of portions of these lymph nodes. The low T2 signal and relative hypoenhancement reflect the presence of fibrotic material caused by hyalinization of these lymph nodes, an important diagnostic feature differentiating a deactivating or old granulomatous process from an early or active granulomatous process, reactive lymphadenopathy, and neoplastic lymphadenopathy. Note that more active sarcoidosis may not be sufficiently hyalinized to show this sign.

distinction of an acquired or congenital cyst with proteinaceous content.

### Smooth muscle and fibrous tissue

Relative T2 hypointensity (approximate isointensity to muscle on T2-weighted images) can be a meaningful diagnostic finding, because most mediastinal lesions are overtly T2-hyperintense to muscle.[9] T2 hypointensity can be found in lesions containing hemosiderin, smooth muscle, and fibrous tissue.[9,29,30]

The densely packed, water-poor, actin and myosin–rich smooth muscle fibers of an esophageal leiomyoma can readily differentiate this benign lesion from a foregut duplication cyst or primary esophageal malignancy (**Fig. 10**). Similarly, the most common fibrous variant of solitary fibrous tumors, chronic fibrosing mediastinitis, and immunoglobulin (Ig) G4–related sclerosing mediastinal lesions can result in T2-hypointense signal

isoattenuating prevascular mediastinal lymphadenopathy, with persistent abnormal soft tissue in this region. ECG-gated DIR T2-weighted MR image (*C*) shows markedly T2-hypointense soft tissue. In-phase (*D*) and opposed-phase (*E*) T1-weighted MR images with ROIs (*F, G*) reveal no loss of signal to indicate the presence of microscopic fat/thymic hyperplasia. The low T2 signal of this tissue reflects the presence of fibrotic tissue and indicates a favorable response to therapy, as opposed to recurrent lymphoma.

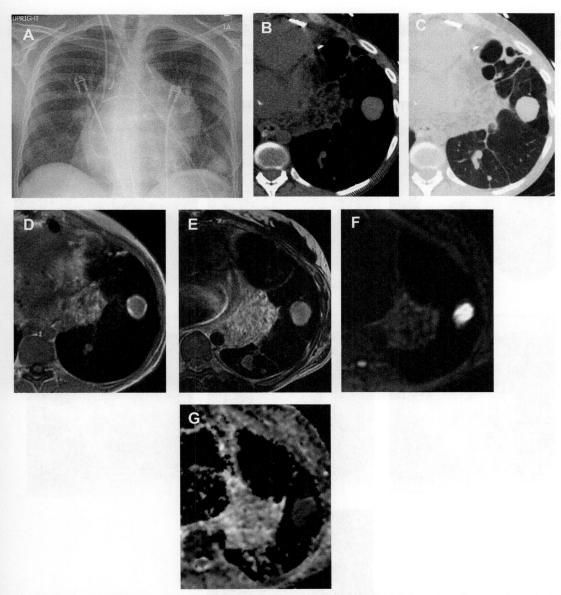

**Fig. 14.** Complementary information provided by DWI and ADC. Diffusion restriction in a pulmonary hematoma. New nodular opacity identified on radiography (*A*) of a 29-year-old woman being evaluated for a second ortho-topic heart transplant. Unenhanced axial CT scans of the chest in soft tissue (*B*) and lung (*C*) windows reveal the radiographic abnormality to be an indeterminate, well-circumscribed, isoattenuating lingular nodule along the anterior margin of the major fissure. There was clinical concern for posttransplant lymphoproliferative disease, which would disqualify her from the transplant list, but interventionists were hesitant because the morbidity and mortality risk of biopsy was high. Axial in-phase T1-weighted (*D*) and radially acquired, axial T2-weighted fast spin-echo MR images (*E*) show internal T1-isointense and T2-hyperintense signal, with a thin rind of periph-eral T1 hyperintensity and greater T2 hyperintensity. IV gadolinium could not be administered at the time because of renal insufficiency. Axial images with diffusion-weighting (*F*) and the corresponding ADC map (*G*) show hyperintense signal on DWI and markedly hypointense signal on the ADC map, indicating restricted diffu-sion of water in this lesion. Constellation of MR imaging findings was compatible with a densely packed, orga-nized hematoma, which subsequently resolved on follow-up imaging. A pulmonary abscess could also yield this appearance; however, there was no evidence of pulmonary infection adjacent to the lingular mass and no clinical evidence of infection. She was therefore able to remain on the transplant list and ultimately underwent a second cardiac transplant.

(**Fig. 11**) secondary to tightly packed, water-poor collagen fibers.[31,32] The presence of patchy T2 hypointensity within lymph nodes, even before their calcification, can indicate hyalinization caused by treated lymphoma (**Fig. 12**) or old granulomatous disease such as sarcoid[29] (**Fig. 13**). Nontreated lymphoma and other noncalcified lymphadenopathy is T2 hyperintense.

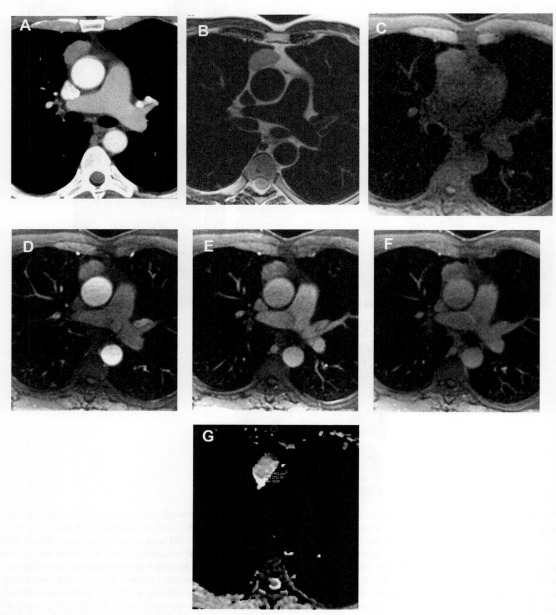

**Fig. 15.** Diagnostic value of DCE and ADC map. Homogeneous enhancement and ADC value of low-risk thymoma. Contrast-enhanced axial CT of the chest (*A*) revealed an intermediate-attenuation mass in the right thymic bed. Axial ECG-gated DIR T2-weighted MR image (*B*) reveals a mildly lobulated T2-hyperintense mass in the right thymic bed. Axial precontrast (*C*) and postcontrast (*D–F*) fat-saturated T1-weighted MR images show a T1-isointense mass with homogeneous enhancement at 20 seconds (*D*), 1 minute (*E*), and 5 minutes (*F*) after gadolinium administration with rapid time-to-peak enhancement at 1 minute, and relative washout at 5 minutes. Supplemental ADC map (*G*) reveals an ADC value of $1.7 \times 10^{-3}$ mm$^2$/s. The lesion morphology, brisk homogeneous enhancement pattern, as well as ADC value greater than $1.25 \times 10^{-3}$ mm$^2$/s suggests a low-risk thymoma. Surgical resection confirmed the diagnosis of thymoma, type AB.

## Diffusion-weighted imaging and apparent diffusion coefficient

DWI and the ADC map it creates evaluate the extent to which water molecules are free to move or are restricted within a lesion. Although more susceptible to artifacts in the thorax because of the multiple air–soft tissue interfaces and

cardiorespiratory motion, this sequence can be helpful in delineating benign and malignant lesions. Breath-hold or respiratory-triggered technique is critical to obtaining a credible ADC map. In general, highly cellular, malignant tissue has a greater propensity to restrict the motion of water molecules. Important benign exceptions to this

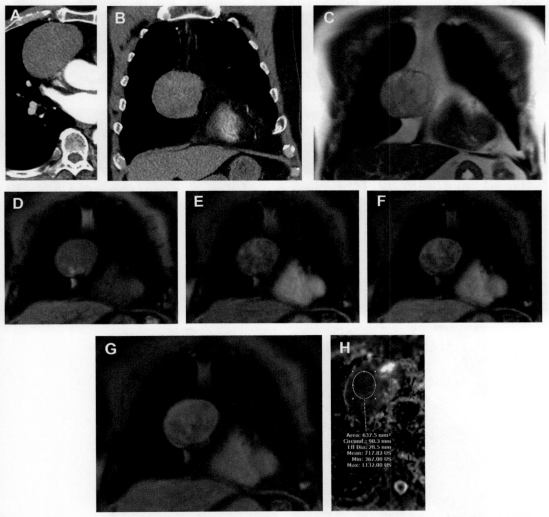

**Fig. 16.** Diagnostic value of DCE and ADC map. Heterogeneous enhancement and ADC value of a more aggressive thymic neoplasm. A positive tuberculin skin test prompted a chest radiograph and subsequent contrast-enhanced CT of the chest of a 58-year-old man with axial (*A*) and coronal (*B*) images revealing an indeterminate soft tissue mass in the prevascular mediastinum. Coronal single-shot fast spin-echo (SSFSE) MR image (*C*) shows a heterogeneously T2-hyperintense mass in the right thymic bed. Coronal precontrast 3D ultrafast GRE, fat-saturated, T1-weighted MR image (*D*) reveals the internal content of this mass to be isointense to skeletal muscle, with foci of hyperintense signal. Postcontrast fat-saturated T1-weighted DCE images (*E–G*) performed at 20 seconds (*E*), 1 minute (*F*), and 5 minutes (*G*) after IV gadolinium administration reveal progressive, heterogenous enhancement, peaking at 5 minutes. ADC map image (*H*) reveals an ADC value of $0.72 \times 10^{-3}$ mm$^2$/s. The lesion morphology, heterogeneous and sustained enhancement pattern, as well as ADC value less than $1.25 \times 10^{-3}$ mm$^2$/s suggest a more aggressive thymic neoplasm. Surgical resection confirmed the mass to be a thymic neuroendocrine tumor. Note that the DCE patterns of this rare tumor may vary, depending on grade and content.

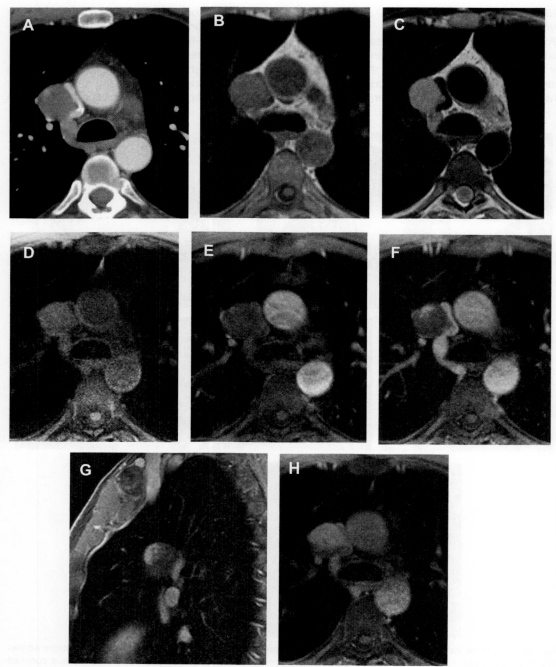

**Fig. 17.** Diagnostic value of DCE imaging. Indeterminate right visceral mediastinal mass protruding into the superior vena cava (SVC) on CT; hemangioma on MR imaging. Contrast-enhanced axial CT of the chest (*A*) reveals a round, well-circumscribed, 30-HU mass compressing or involving the SVC. The mass is of homogeneous attenuation, aside from a focal, hyperattenuating, right anterolateral, peripheral component. The differential diagnosis is broad. Axial in-phase GRE T1-weighted (*B*), ECG-gated DIR T2-weighted (*C*), and precontrast (*D*) and postcontrast (*E–H*) ultrafast 3D GRE MR images reveal the mass to be T1-isointense and markedly T2-hyperintense and to show early, peripheral nodular enhancement (*E*) at 20 seconds, with progressive fill-in over time (*F,* 1 minute axial; *G,* 3 minutes sagittal; and *H,* 5 minutes axial postcontrast MR images). These findings are virtually pathognomonic for a hemangioma. Note that, as in the liver, mediastinal hemangiomas can also show other patterns of enhancement. (*From* Ackman JB. Thoracic MRI: Technique and Approach to Diagnosis. In Shepard JAO: Thoracic Imaging, The Requisites. Philadelphia: Elsevier, p 61-87; with permission.)

general concept are congealed hematomas and abscesses, which, on account of their thickened texture, can also be restricted (**Fig. 14**). This concept can be used to help differentiate benign from malignant lesions throughout the mediastinum, as shown by Gümüştaş and colleagues,[33] using an ADC cutoff of $1.39 \times 10^{-3}$ mm/s with a sensitivity of 95% and specificity of 87%. Additional investigations have applied this concept to primary mediastinal tumors as well as malignant lymph nodes.[34–37] For example, Abdel Razek and colleagues[34] found a cutoff ADC value less than 1.25 and $1.22 \times 10^{-3}$ mm²/s to be helpful in differentiating low-risk thymoma from high-risk thymoma and thymic carcinoma, respectively (**Figs. 15** and **16**).

### Dynamic contrast enhancement

Evaluation of DCE using IV gadolinium and precontrast and postcontrast, ultrafast GRE, fat-

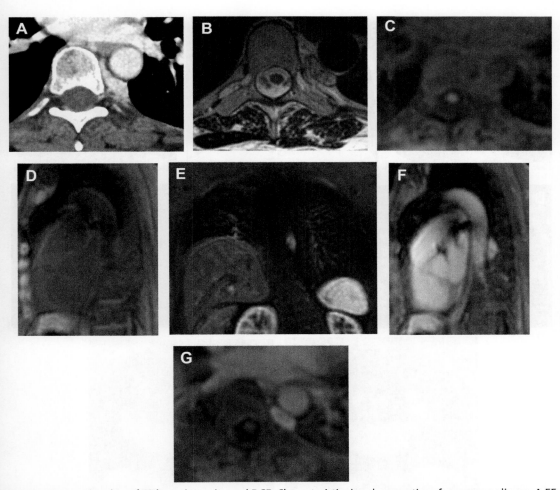

**Fig. 18.** Diagnostic value of T2 hyperintensity and DCE. Characteristic signal properties of a paraganglioma. A 55-year-old woman with germline mutation of the succinate dehydrogenase enzyme-subunit B and prior resection of neck and abdominal paragangliomas. An abnormal iodine-123 meta-iodobenzylguanidine scan prompted cross-sectional imaging. Contrast-enhanced axial CT of the chest reveals an avidly enhancing left paravertebral mass overlying the neck of the adjacent rib (*A*) corresponding to the scintigraphic abnormality. 2D spin-echo T2-weighted MR image without fat saturation (*B*) reveals the mass to be markedly T2-hyperintense to muscle, as is typical of paragangliomas. Axial (*C*) and sagittal (*D*) precontrast and coronal 20 second, sagittal 3-minute, and axial 5-minute postcontrast (*E–G*) fat-saturated T1-weighted MR images show a T1-isointense mass, oriented longitudinally in the craniocaudal dimension, with rapid, vigorous enhancement at 20 seconds, peaking at 3 minutes. The location, morphology, and MR imaging signal and enhancement pattern of this mass are characteristic of a paraganglioma. Note that the salt-and-pepper appearance of paragangliomas is not universally present and is often not seen in small mediastinal paragangliomas.

saturated T1-weighted imaging is helpful for further characterization of mediastinal lesions when noncontrast imaging is inconclusive. The temporal enhancement pattern, heterogeneity versus homogeneity of enhancement, and presence or absence of cystic change and necrosis can be very informative. Thin, smooth capsular or wall enhancement is a reassuring finding, because it usually represents the thin epithelial or pseudoepithelial layer of tissue found in certain lesions (acquired or congenital thymic and foregut duplication cysts). Alternatively, the presence of enhancing, irregular wall thickening, thick or irregular septations, and/or mural nodularity within an otherwise cystic lesion increases the likelihood of malignancy, although it does not ensure it (see **Fig. 3**).[38,39]

Solid lesional enhancement, and, further, its homogeneity or lack thereof, and degree of enhancement can also increase diagnostic specificity. The

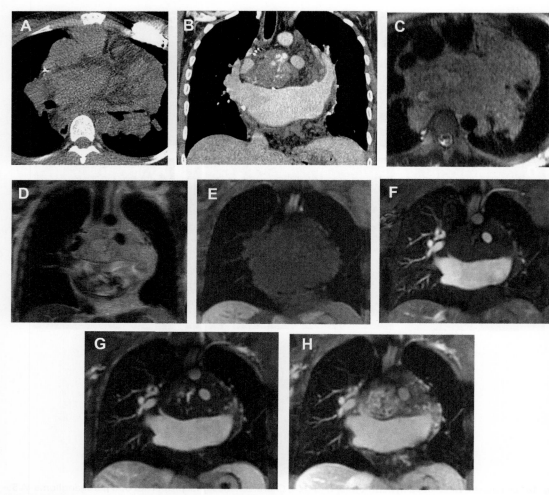

**Fig. 19.** Diagnostic value of DCE. Progressive enhancement of lymphatic malformation in a 35-year-old woman with prior orthotopic heart transplant and several weeks of fevers. Unenhanced axial CT of the chest (A) shows a multilobulated visceral mediastinal, partially intrapericardial, mass that showed areas of enhancement on coronal postcontrast CT. (B) A lymphoproliferative process was favored. Axial (C) and coronal (D) SSFSE T2W MR images reveal T2-hyperintense, multilocular tissue throughout the visceral mediastinum, insinuating between cardiovascular structures. Coronal precontrast 3D ultrafast GRE, fat-saturated T1-weighted MR image (E) reveals the internal content of this multilocular tissue to be hypointense to skeletal muscle. Postcontrast fat-saturated T1-weighted MR images (F–H) performed at 20 seconds (F), 1 minute (G), and 5 minutes (H) after IV gadolinium administration reveal heterogenous enhancement and progressive fill-in of the lesion consistent with a lymphatic malformation, attributed to iatrogenic disruption of mediastinal lymphatics during cardiac transplant. Note that it can take up to 10 minutes for lymphatic malformations to fill or enhance with IV contrast.

fairly homogeneous enhancement of a low-risk thymoma may help distinguish it from the more heterogeneous enhancement of a high-risk thymoma, thymic carcinoma, and thymic carcinoid[40–42] (see **Figs. 15** and **16**). The presence of enhancement within a lesion not only highlights its solid, cellular components but can also, at times, be used as a surrogate for disease activity and may be used to monitor response to therapy. For example, active mediastinal lymphoma more

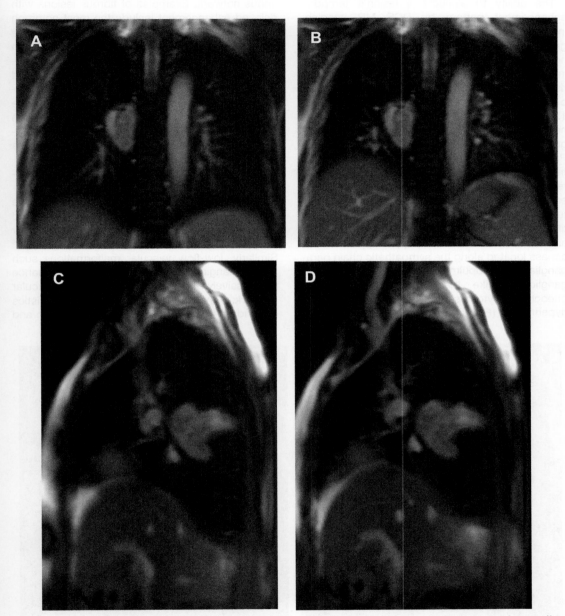

**Fig. 20.** MR sniff test employed to ascertain whether a paravertebral soft tissue mass is fixed to the chest wall or mobile during free-breathing. Coronal and sagittal inspiratory (*A, C*) and expiratory (*B, D*) SSFP MR images acquired during tidal breathing and sniffing show a heterogeneous signal intensity, mushroom-shaped mass in the paravertebral mediastinum, with a component extending toward, but not clearly arising from, the right T7-8 neural foramina. The differential diagnosis includes a solitary fibrous tumor (which typically arises from visceral pleura) and a schwannoma. The mass remains stationary throughout respiration, because it is fixed to the spine. A noninvasive solitary fibrous tumor arising from the visceral pleura would be expected to move, relative to the chest wall, during free breathing. Surgical resection confirmed the diagnosis of a schwannoma. Please refer to the coronal (Video 1) and sagittal (Video 2) videos of this MR sniff test.

avidly enhances than treated lymphoma.[43–46] Similarly, enhancement characteristics of mediastinal lymph nodes can also be informative in other lymphoproliferative processes and metastatic disease.[47–49]

The ability to evaluate a lesion's temporal enhancement pattern by DCE MR imaging, including its time-to-peak enhancement and degree of washout, may further contribute to diagnostic specificity. Enhancement kinetics can be informative in the setting of thymoma, with low-risk thymomas showing more rapid time-to-peak-enhancement kinetics (typically around 1.3 minutes) than high-risk thymoma, thymic carcinoma, and lymphoma, which tend to show more gradual enhancement out to 3 to 5 minutes.[50,51] Paraganglioma is the prototypical mediastinal mass of early peak enhancement and delayed retention of contrast, with characteristic brisk enhancement attributed to its hypervascular nature, sometimes (although rarely in the mediastinum) with visible intratumoral vessels depicted as flow voids or a salt-and-pepper appearance in a mass located along the sympathetic chain paraganglia and aortopulmonary paraganglia.[9,52] Paragangliomas, like their adrenal counterparts, pheochromocytomas, are classically very T2-hyperintense (**Fig. 17**).

Delayed time-to-peak-enhancement kinetics can be seen in fibrous lesions. Delayed peak enhancement in fibrotic lesions results from the diminutive vascular supply or endothelial disruption at the capillary level among the dense collagenous network. Examples of fibrous lesions with delayed enhancement include the most common variant of solitary fibrous tumors (fibrous) of the mediastinum and pleura and hyalinized lymph nodes in the setting of sarcoidosis, chronic fibrosing mediastinitis, treated lymphoma, and old tuberculosis (see **Fig. 13**). Tuberculous lymphadenitis can be informative in this regard because enhancement characteristics of involved lymph nodes evolve throughout the disease process during the different stages of necrosis and granuloma formation.[53]

Hemangiomas and other low-flow vascular malformations are rare in the mediastinum. Hemangiomas in the mediastinum show similar variable enhancement patterns to those in the liver and can show discontinuous peripheral nodular enhancement with progressive fill-in (**Fig. 18**).[54] Similarly, low-flow vascular malformations such as lymphangiomas or angiomatosis may enhance progressively because of their dysplastic vascular network; individual imaging characteristics depend on combination or ratio of lymphatic and

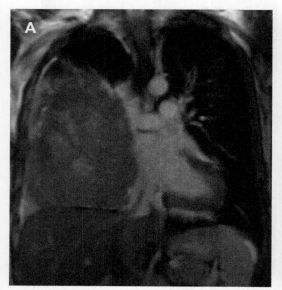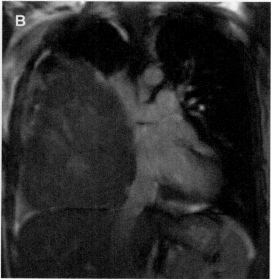

**Fig. 21.** MR sniff test employed for phrenic nerve/diaphragmatic function assessment in the setting of a large thymic squamous cell carcinoma with invasive components in the right prevascular mediastinum. Coronal inspiratory (*A*) and expiratory (*B*) free-breathing SSFP MR images show a large, heterogeneous signal intensity mass extending from the suprahilar right prevascular mediastinum to the level of the diaphragm, spanning a segment of the anticipated course of the right phrenic nerve. On inspiration, the left hemidiaphragm appropriately moves caudally. On expiration, the left hemidiaphragm appropriately moves cephalad. However, the right hemidiaphragm moves cranially or paradoxically during inspiration, indicating right hemidiaphragmatic paralysis secondary to involvement of the right phrenic nerve by tumor. Please refer to the video (Video 3) of this MR sniff test.

vascular components (**Fig. 19**). Without delayed imaging beyond 5 minutes, the enhancement of some lymphangiomas may not be appreciable.[55–58]

### Relationship to adjacent structures

The superior tissue contrast afforded by MR imaging enables further definition of the borders of a given lesion. This definition can be beneficial when determining the site of origin of a particular mass or evaluating its resectability. The ability of MR imaging to establish invasion of a lesion into adjacent tissue plays an important role in operative (or nonoperative) planning of resection of certain lesions, as well as prognostic staging of bronchogenic and esophageal malignancies.[59,60]

Dynamic cine sequences performed during free breathing and sniffing allow discernment of whether a lesion is mobile in relation to the adjacent tissue or stuck to it, whether caused by invasion across tissue planes, inflammation, or fibrous reaction. As discussed previously, this technique may allow determination of the site of origin of a mass, as in the case of a fibrous tumor of the pleura, by ascertaining movement or sliding of this typically visceral pleural lesion relative to the chest wall, or in the case of a stationary paravertebral schwannoma affixed to the chest wall (**Fig. 20**). This technique may also be helpful in establishing invasion of a mediastinal mass into adjacent mediastinal structures (**Fig. 21**), pleura, or lung, or invasion of a lung cancer into the mediastinum, superior sulcus, or chest wall.

### Management and follow-up

Because MR imaging adds diagnostic specificity beyond that of CT and fluorodeoxyglucose PET/CT, it can often prevent further follow-up imaging and unnecessary biopsy or resection. Occasionally, a mediastinal lesion remains indeterminate after MR imaging evaluation. In such cases, surveillance by serial MR imaging reduces the compounded ionizing radiation exposure that would be delivered by CT surveillance and provides the additional benefit of more comprehensive tissue characterization and detection of subtle interval change, including increased mural nodularity and septations, at each time point.[61] Examples of lesions that may warrant follow-up include cystic thymic lesions with mild wall thickening greater than or equal to 3 mm and/or minimal mural nodularity/fine septations, because these lesions can be inflammatory and do not always represent rare cystic thymomas (see **Fig. 3**). Foregut duplication cysts can also be followed to assess their growth rate and potential to compress vital mediastinal structures.[1,2] The

lack of ionizing radiation also makes MR an excellent modality to follow indeterminate lesions and malignancy in young, pregnant, and radiation-adverse patients and in patients at increased risk for radiation-induced cancers. An abbreviated protocol can be implemented for surveillance, sometimes without IV contrast, when a lesion has been previously characterized.

### SUMMARY

Thoracic MR imaging plays an important role in evaluation of patients with mediastinal lesions. Thoughtful protocol design tailored to the clinical question can significantly affect the diagnostic evaluation and alter patient management. Knowledge of the role of MR imaging for these patients and understanding the implications of specific imaging characteristics can improve patient care and add immense value.

### CLINICS CARE POINTS

- The superior soft tissue contrast and tissue characterization properties of MR imaging often allow diagnosis of indeterminate mediastinal lesions on CT.
- Identification of T2 hypointensity within a mediastinal lesion often drastically narrows its differential diagnosis, given that most mediastinal lesions are T2-hyperintense.
- Chemical shift MR imaging allows confident determination of the presence of microscopic fat within a lesion, whether by qualitative observation or SII and CSR calculation.
- Dynamic contrast-enhanced MR imaging allows temporal evaluation of enhancement characteristics, adding important diagnostic information without ionizing radiation exposure.
- Evaluation of the ADC map helps differentiate benign from malignant lesions throughout the mediastinum.

### SUPPLEMENTARY DATA

Supplementary data related to this article can be found online at https://doi.org/10.1016/j.rcl.2020.11.001.

### REFERENCES

1. Ackman JB, Verzosa S, Kovach AE, et al. High rate of unnecessary thymectomy and its cause. Can computed tomography distinguish thymoma, lymphoma, thymic hyperplasia, and thymic cysts? Eur J Radiol 2015;84(3):524–33.

2. Ackman JB, Gaissert HA, Lanuti M, et al. Impact of nonvascular thoracic MR imaging on the clinical decision making of thoracic surgeons: a 2-year prospective study. Radiology 2016;280(2):464–74.

3. Thierry-Chef I, Dabin J, Friberg E, et al. Assessing organ doses from paediatric CT scans—A novel approach for an epidemiology study (the EPI-CT Study). Int J Environ Res Public Health 2013;10(2):717–28.

4. Brenner DJ, Elliston CD, Hall EJ, et al. Estimated risks of radiation-induced fatal cancer from pediatric CT. AJR Am J Roentgenol 2001;176(2):289–96.

5. Niemann T, Colas L, Roser HW, et al. Estimated risk of radiation-induced cancer from paediatric chest CT: two-year cohort study. Pediatr Radiol 2015;45(3):329–36.

6. Pearce MS, Salotti JA, Little MP, et al. Radiation exposure from CT scans in childhood and subsequent risk of leukaemia and brain tumours: a retrospective cohort study. Lancet 2012;380(9840):499–505.

7. Smith-Bindman R, Lipson J, Marcus R, et al. Radiation dose associated with common computed tomography examinations and the associated lifetime attributable risk of cancer. Arch Intern Med 2009;169(22):2078–86.

8. Sodickson A, Baeyens PF, Andriole KP, et al. Recurrent CT, cumulative radiation exposure, and associated radiation-induced cancer risks from CT of adults. Radiology 2009;251(1):175–84.

9. Ackman JB. MR imaging of mediastinal masses. Magn Reson Imaging Clin N Am 2015;23(2):141–64.

10. Lee SH, Hur J, Kim YJ, et al. Additional value of dual-energy CT to differentiate between benign and malignant mediastinal tumors: an initial experience. Eur J Radiol 2013;82(11):2043–9.

11. Otrakji A, Digumarthy SR, Lo Gullo R, et al. Dual-energy CT: spectrum of thoracic abnormalities. Radiographics 2016;36(1):38–52.

12. Megibow AJ, Chandarana H, Hindman NM. Increasing the precision of CT measurements with dual-energy scanning. Radiology 2014;272(3):618–21.

13. Ackman JB, Nitiwarangkul C, Mercaldo SF. Extent of intraprotocol and intersite variability of thoracic magnetic resonance acquisition times at a large quaternary institution: MR technologist insights as to its causes. J Thorac Imaging 2019;34(6):356–61.

14. Raptis CA, McWilliams SR, Ratkowski KL, et al. Mediastinal and pleural MR imaging: practical approach for daily practice. Radiographics 2018;38(1):37–55.

15. Ackman JB. A practical guide to nonvascular thoracic magnetic resonance imaging. J Thorac Imaging 2014;29(1):17–29.

16. Raptis CA, Ludwig DR, Hammer MM, et al. Building blocks for thoracic MRI: challenges, sequences, and protocol design. J Magn Reson Imaging 2019;50(3):682–701.

17. Ackman JB, Kovacina B, Carter BW, et al. Sex difference in normal thymic appearance in adults 20–30 years of age. Radiology 2013. https://doi.org/10.1148/radiol.13121104.

18. Baron RL, Lee JK, Sagel SS, et al. Computed tomography of the normal thymus. Radiology 1982;142(1):121.

19. Ackman JB, Wu CC. MRI of the thymus. AJR Am J Roentgenol 2011;197(1):W15–20.

20. Inaoka T, Takahashi K, Mineta M, et al. Thymic hyperplasia and thymus gland tumors: differentiation with chemical shift MR Imaging. Radiology 2007;243(3):869–76.

21. Takahashi K, Inaoka T, Murakami N, et al. Characterization of the normal and hyperplastic thymus on chemical-shift MR imaging. AJR Am J Roentgenol 2003;180(5):1265–9.

22. Priola AM, Priola SM, Ciccone G, et al. Differentiation of rebound and lymphoid thymic hyperplasia from anterior mediastinal tumors with dual-echo chemical-shift MR imaging in adulthood: reliability of the chemical-shift ratio and signal intensity index. Radiology 2015;274(1):238–49.

23. Ackman JB, Mino-Kenudson M, Morse CR. Nonsuppressing normal thymus on chemical shift magnetic resonance imaging in a young woman. J Thorac Imaging 2012;27(6):W196–8.

24. Priola AM, Priola SM, Gned D, et al. Nonsuppressing normal thymus on chemical-shift MR imaging and anterior mediastinal lymphoma: differentiation with diffusion-weighted MR imaging by using the apparent diffusion coefficient. Eur Radiol 2018;28(4):1427–37.

25. Priola AM, Gned D, Marci V, et al. Diffusion-weighted MRI in a case of nonsuppressing rebound thymic hyperplasia on chemical-shift MRI. Jpn J Radiol 2015;33(3):158–63.

26. Phung T, Nguyen T, Tran D, et al. A thymic hyperplasia case without suppressing on chemical shift magnetic resonance imaging. Case Rep Radiol 2018;2018:1–4.

27. McInnis MC, Flores EJ, Shepard J-AO, et al. Pitfalls in the imaging and interpretation of benign thymic lesions: how thymic MRI can help. AJR Am J Roentgenol 2016;206(1):W1–8.

28. Bradley WG. MR appearance of hemorrhage in the brain. Radiology 1993;189(1):15–26. Bradley WG, ed.

29. Chung JH, Cox CW, Forssen AV, et al. The dark lymph node sign on magnetic resonance imaging: a novel finding in patients with sarcoidosis. J Thorac Imaging 2014;29(2):125–9.

30. Leyendecker JR. Practical guide to abdominal & pelvic MRI. 2nd edition. Philadelphia: Wolters Kluwer Health/Lippincott Williams & Wilkins; 2011.

31. Wilhelm A, Jolles HI, Krishna M. Anterior mediastinal desmoid tumor with CT and MR imaging. J Thorac Imaging 2007;22(3):252–5.

32. Wallace ZS, Perugino C, Matza M, et al. Immuno-globulin G4–related disease. Clin Chest Med 2019; 40(3):583–97.

33. Gümüştaş S, İnan N, Sarisoy HT, et al. Malignant versus benign mediastinal lesions: quantitative assessment with diffusion weighted MR imaging. Eur Radiol 2011;21(11):2255–60.

34. Razek AA, Elmorsy A, Elshafey M, et al. Assessment of mediastinal tumors with diffusion-weighted single-shot echo-planar MRI. J Magn Reson Imaging 2009; 30(3):535–40.

35. Razek AAKA, Ashmalla GA. Assessment of paraspinal neurogenic tumors with diffusion-weighted MR imaging. Eur Spine J 2018;27(4):841.

36. Nomori H, Mori T, Ikeda K, et al. Diffusion-weighted magnetic resonance imaging can be used in place of positron emission tomography for N staging of non–small cell lung cancer with fewer false-positive results. J Thorac Cardiovasc Surg 2008;135(4):816–22.

37. Abdel Razek AAK, Khairy M, Nada N. Diffusion-weighted MR imaging in thymic epithelial tumors: correlation with World Health Organization Classification and clinical staging. Radiology 2014;273(1):268–75.

38. Jeung M-Y, Gasser B, Gangi A, et al. Imaging of cystic masses of the mediastinum. Radiographics 2002;22(suppl_1):S79–93.

39. Madan R, Ratanaprasatporn L, Ratanaprasatporn L, et al. Cystic mediastinal masses and the role of MRI. Clin Imaging 2018;50:68–77.

40. Carter BW, Benveniste MFK, Truong MT, et al. State of the art. Magn Reson Imaging Clin N Am 2015; 23(2):165–77.

41. Shimamoto A, Ashizawa K, Kido Y, et al. CT and MRI findings of thymic carcinoid. Br J Radiol 2017; 90(1071):20150341.

42. Restrepo CS, Pandit M, Rojas IC, et al. Imaging findings of expansile lesions of the thymus. Curr Probl Diagn Radiol 2005;34(1):22–34.

43. Rahmouni A, Divine M, Lepage E, et al. Mediastinal lymphoma: quantitative changes in gadolinium enhancement at MR imaging after treatment. Radiology 2001;219(3):621–8.

44. Hill M, Cunningham D, MacVicar D, et al. Role of magnetic resonance imaging in predicting relapse in residual masses after treatment of lymphoma. J Clin Oncol 1993;11(11):2273–8.

45. Devizzi L, Maffioli L, Bonfante V, et al. Comparison of gallium scan, computed tomography, and magnetic resonance in patients with mediastinal Hodgkin's disease. Ann Oncol 1997;8:S53–6.

46. Gasparini MD, Balzarini L, Castellani MR, et al. Current role of gallium scan and magnetic resonance imaging in the management of mediastinal Hodgkin lymphoma. Cancer 1993;72(2):577–82.

47. Choi SH, Moon W. Contrast-enhanced MR imaging of lymph nodes in cancer patients. Korean J Radiol 2010;11(4):383–94.

48. Hasegawa I, Eguchi K, Kohda E, et al. Pulmonary hilar lymph nodes in lung cancer: assessment with 3D-dynamic contrast-enhanced MR imaging. Eur J Radiol 2003;45(2):129–34.

49. Pannu HK, Wang K-P, Borman TL, et al. MR imaging of mediastinal lymph nodes: evaluation using a superparamagnetic contrast agent. J Magn Reson Imaging 2000;12(6):899–904.

50. Sakai S, Murayama S, Soeda H, et al. Differential diagnosis between thymoma and non-thymoma by dynamic MR imaging. Acta Radiol 2002;43(3): 262–8.

51. Marom EM. Advances in thymoma imaging. J Thorac Imaging 2013;28(2):69–83.

52. Balcombe J, Torigian DA, Kim W, et al. Cross-sectional imaging of paragangliomas of the aortic body and other thoracic branchiomeric paraganglia. AJR Am J Roentgenol 2007;188(4): 1054–8.

53. Moon WK, Im JG, Yu IK, et al. Mediastinal tuberculous lymphadenitis: MR imaging appearance with clinicopathologic correlation. AJR Am J Roentgenol 1996;166(1):21–5.

54. Semelka RC, Brown ED, Ascher SM, et al. Hepatic hemangiomas: a multi-institutional study of appearance on T2-weighted and serial gadolinium-enhanced gradient-echo MR images. Radiology 1994;192(2):401–6. Semelka RC, ed.

55. Donnelly LF, Adams DM, Bisset GS. Vascular malformations and hemangiomas. AJR Am J Roentgenol 2000;174(3):597-608.

56. Ohgiya Y, Hashimoto T, Gokan T, et al. Dynamic MRI for distinguishing high-flow from low-flow peripheral vascular malformations. AJR Am J Roentgenol 2005; 185(5):1131–7.

57. White CL, Olivieri B, Restrepo R, et al. Low-flow vascular malformation pitfalls: from clinical examination to practical imaging evaluation—part 1, lymphatic malformation mimickers. AJR Am J Roentgenol 2016;206(5):940–51.

58. Olivieri B, White CL, Restrepo R, et al. Low-flow vascular malformation pitfalls: from clinical examination to practical imaging evaluation—part 2, venous malformation mimickers. AJR Am J Roentgenol 2016;206(5):952–62.

59. Ohno Y, Koyama H, Ho YL, et al. Magnetic Resonance Imaging (MRI) and Positron Emission Tomography (PET)/MRI for lung cancer staging. J Thorac Imaging 2016;31(4):215–27.

60. Riddell AM, Hillier J, Brown G, et al. Potential of surface-coil MRI for staging of esophageal cancer. AJR Am J Roentgenol 2006;187(5):1280–7.

61. Ackman JB, Chung JH, Walker C, et al. ACR Appropriateness Criteria Imaging of Mediastinal Masses. Journal of American College of Radiology 2020. Available at: https://acsearch.acr.org/docs/3157912/Narrative/.

# Potential Pitfalls in Imaging of the Mediastinum

Orly Goitein, MD[a],*, Mylene T. Truong, MD[b], Elena Bekker, MD[a,c],
Edith M. Marom, MD[c]

## KEYWORDS

• Thoracic • Mediastinum • CT • MR imaging • Pitfalls

## KEY POINTS

• Advances in computed tomography technology allow visualization of normal anatomic structures and variants in greater detail, which can be misinterpreted as pathology.
• If a mediastinal mass is suspected to be cystic, MR imaging adds value by demonstrating its fluid content and is helpful to differentiate benign from malignant disease.
• An awareness of the spectrum of the potential pitfalls of mediastinal imaging and artifacts related to flow, motion, and cardiac pulsations is important for accurate interpretation.
• Flow artifacts can be resolved by obtaining a delayed venous scan.
• Artifacts owing to cardiac motion can be mitigated by using electrocardiographic gating.

## INTRODUCTION

A computed tomography (CT) scan of the chest is the modality of choice for evaluating many suspected or known thoracic abnormalities involving the lungs and mediastinum. CT scans are widely available with a relatively quick acquisition time and allows for accurate and reproducible images of the mediastinum, its contents, and any associated abnormalities. Advances in multidetector CT technology, with improved temporal and spatial resolution, allow for better delineation of mediastinal structures. However, the high resolution of a CT scan also results in the routine visualization of normal anatomic structures and anatomic variants, which can be confused with pathology, as well as benign lesions that may mimic malignant neoplasms.

A CT scan may be performed for a variety of clinical scenarios, both in the acute and ambulatory settings.[1] Ideally, the CT protocol is optimized and tailored to answer a specific clinical question or concern. However, many mediastinal abnormalities are discovered incidentally, and a CT scan of the chest performed in the routine fashion may be insufficient for the purposes of developing a focused differential diagnosis. Some artifacts induced by technique may simulate pathology, and additional evaluation with electrocardiographic (ECG)-gated cardiac CT scans, MR imaging, or a PET/CT scan with fluorodeoxyglucose (FDG) may add value. An awareness of the potential pitfalls in assessing the mediastinum on imaging studies and effective solutions to mitigate these problematic issues is necessary to ensure an accurate interpretation by radiologists. The

[a] Department of Diagnostic Imaging, Division of Cardiovascular Imaging, The Chaim Sheba Medical Center (affiliated with Tel Aviv University), Derech Sheba 2, Ramat Gan, Israel; [b] Department of Diagnostic Imaging, Division of Thoracic Imaging, University of Texas MD Anderson Cancer Center, 1515 Holcombe Boulevard, Houston, TX 77030, USA; [c] Department of Diagnostic Imaging, Division of Thoracic Imaging, The Chaim Sheba Medical Center (affiliated with Tel Aviv University), Derech Sheba 2, Ramat Gan, Israel
* Corresponding author. The Chaim Sheba Medical Center, Derech Sheba 2, Ramat Gan, Israel.
E-mail address: orly.goitein@sheba.health.gov.il

Radiol Clin N Am 59 (2021) 279–290
https://doi.org/10.1016/j.rcl.2020.11.003
0033-8389/21/© 2020 Elsevier Inc. All rights reserved.

purpose of this review is to highlight and discuss the potential pitfalls in the imaging of the mediastinum.

## CYSTIC STRUCTURES

Cystic or fluid-containing structures are commonly encountered in all compartments of the mediastinum, and may represent normal anatomy (such as fluid in the pericardial recesses), cysts (such as thymic or bronchogenic cyst), or cystic neoplasms (such as cystic thymoma). It is important to differentiate cystic neoplasms from benign lesions and normal anatomic structures to ensure appropriate intervention and avoid delays in treatment planning.

In the oncologic setting, one of the most commonly encountered mediastinal anatomic pitfalls relates to pericardial recesses mimicking lymphadenopathy. The pericardium is composed of an outer fibrous component and an inner serous component, which itself has an inner visceral layer, adherent to the heart and great vessels, and an outer parietal layer, which lines the fibrous pericardium. The pericardial space normally contains approximately 15 to 30 mL of fluid between the visceral and parietal layers of the serous pericardium. There are reflections of serous pericardium between the great vessels and at the base of the heart. Physiologic amounts of fluid in these pericardial reflections may vary between imaging studies obtained at different time points. Typical imaging features of fluid-filled pericardial sinuses

and recesses include fluid attenuation, contiguity with other pericardial spaces, and no mass effect on adjacent structures. Multiplanar reformations are particularly helpful in demonstrating the relationship between the pericardial recesses and other mediastinal structures, as well as the contiguity with the rest of the pericardium. A distinctive beak-like appearance is seen as fluid in the pericardial recesses drapes over the neighboring mediastinal structures. Of the various pericardial recesses, the high-riding variant of the superior aortic recess extending cephalad into the right paratracheal region constitutes a potential pitfall in oncologic imaging because it can be confused with lymphadenopathy (**Fig. 1**).[2] Owing to its typical appearance, the use of other imaging modalities to confirm pericardial fluid is usually not necessary. However, when in doubt, MR imaging, with its superior contrast resolution, can show the fluid content with high signal intensity on T2-weighted images, low signal intensity on T1-weighted images, and the lack of enhancement after the administration of intravenous contrast. On CT scans, mediastinal lymphadenopathy manifests as soft tissue lesions with lobular margins that may exert a mass effect on the adjacent structures. Depending on the underlying etiology, enlarged lymph nodes may enhance after the administration of intravenous contrast. FDG PET/CT scans can also help to distinguish lymphadenopathy from the pericardial fluid, with the former demonstrating increased FDG uptake in the

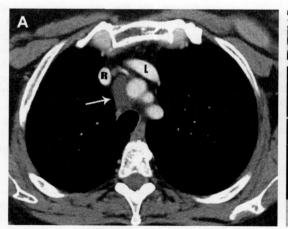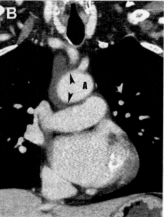

**Fig. 1.** Superior aortic pericardial recess in a 60-year-old woman. (*A*) A contrast-enhanced axial CT scan of the chest at the level of the right (R) and left (L) brachiocephalic veins demonstrates a homogeneous low attenuation fluid collection (*arrow*) between the right brachiocephalic vein and the innominate artery. (*B*) A coronal reformatted contrast-enhanced CT scan of the chest shows fluid adjacent to the brachiocephalic vessels that is contiguous with the superior aortic recess of the transverse sinus draping over the aorta (A) with a beak-like extension (*arrowheads*).

setting of metastatic disease or active infection or inflammation.

Mediastinal cysts are most commonly encountered in the prevascular compartment, typically within the fat anterior to or lateral to the pericardium. Although surgical series have suggested that cysts represent less than 5% of mediastinal masses, a recent multi-institutional study has shown that mediastinal cysts represent 24% of prevascular mediastinal masses.[3] When a cystic lesion is identified in the prevascular mediastinum, the primary role of the radiologist is to differentiate between a benign cyst such as a thymic or pericardial cyst and a cystic thymoma. Thymic cysts are among most common benign thymic lesions and may be either congenital or acquired. Congenital thymic cysts are unilocular, contain clear fluid, and are found incidentally in asymptomatic patients during the first 2 decades of life.[4,5] Acquired thymic cysts may be multilocular and contain heterogeneous fluid indicating a high protein content owing to infection or hemorrhage. Conditions associated with thymic cysts include thymic neoplasms, radiation therapy, thoracotomy, and chest trauma. Unfortunately, thymic cysts often manifest with internal heterogeneous attenuation that cannot be differentiated from cystic neoplasms on CT imaging alone. A common pitfall in the

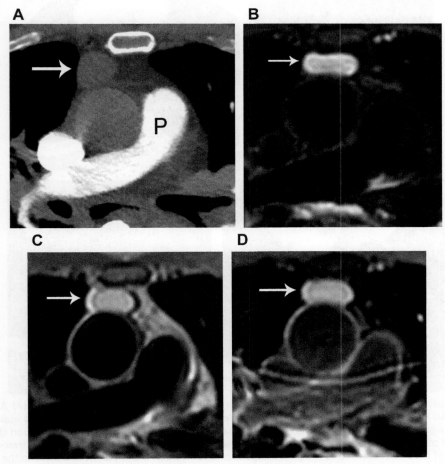

**Fig. 2.** Thymic cyst in a 68-year-old man with shortness of breath. (*A*) A contrast-enhanced axial CT scan of the chest at the level of the pulmonary trunk (P) demonstrates a homogeneous prevascular mediastinal mass measuring 60 Hounsfield units (*arrow*), suspicious for a solid lesion such as thymoma. (*B*) An axial T2-weighted MR image demonstrates homogeneous high signal intensity without thick septations or nodules (*arrow*). (*C*) An axial T1-weighted MR image demonstrates homogeneous high signal intensity in the lesion (*arrow*). (*D*) An axial T1-weighted MR image obtained after the administration of intravenous gadolinium contrast demonstrates no enhancement, thick septations or nodules, characterizing this lesion as a thymic cyst and differentiating it from a cystic thymoma.

evaluation of benign thymic cysts is misinterpretation as solid masses when their attenuation is higher than expected for fluid (higher than 20 Hounsfield units), which may then lead to unnecessary invasive tissue sampling or surgery.[6] To address this issue, MR imaging can be performed to evaluate these lesions, because it is the optimal imaging modality for distinguishing cystic from solid lesions, identifying cystic and/or necrotic lesion components, characterizing cystic lesions as to the presence of septations and mural

nodularity, and distinguishing normal or hyperplastic thymic tissue from neoplasia. Typical characteristics of a thymic cyst on MR imaging include a low signal intensity on T1-weighted images and a uniform high signal intensity on T2-weighted images. After the administration of intravenous contrast, thick, enhancing septations or mural nodularity should be absent (Fig. 2). The presence of these findings should raise concern for a thymic malignancy. A high signal intensity on both T1- and T2-weighted images may represent a cystic lesion

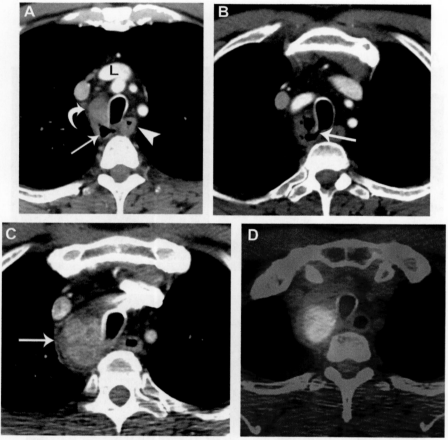

**Fig. 3.** Tracheal diverticulum in a 52-year-old man with undifferentiated sinonasal carcinoma. (*A*) A contrast-enhanced axial CT scan of the chest at the level of the left brachiocephalic vein (L) demonstrates apparent soft tissue in the right paratracheal region mimicking lymphadenopathy (*curved arrow*). However, upon closer scrutiny, a pocket of air (*straight arrow*) separate from the esophagus (*arrowhead*) is noted. (*B*) A contrast-enhanced axial CT scan of the chest cephalad to the prior image demonstrates that the apparent soft tissue in the right paratracheal region actually represents a fluid-filled tracheal diverticulum. Note the air-filled stalk (*arrow*) connecting this lesion to the tracheal lumen. (*C*) A contrast-enhanced axial CT scan of the chest performed 6 days later shows that the tracheal diverticulum (*arrow*) has increased in size, contains more fluid but less air, and enhances heterogeneously. This CT scan was performed 3 days after bronchoscopy in which the diverticulum was brushed and biopsied. (*D*) A fused axial FDG PET/CT scan performed after the bronchoscopy shows increased FDG uptake in the paratracheal lesion that could be misinterpreted as a neoplasm. However, this uptake was due to inflammation from a recent invasive procedure. The tracheal diverticulum decreased in size and FDG avidity on subsequent studies (not shown).

complicated by hemorrhage or infection. To avoid misinterpretation of a thymic malignancy as benign, it is important to pay close attention to the T1-weighted images after intravenous contrast administration, because enhancement is noted in the early dynamic phase in 90% of tumors, and the remaining 10% show enhancement on delayed T1-weighted images.[7]

Tracheal diverticula are outpouchings from the tracheal wall that are lined with ciliated columnar epithelium. They are usually 5 to 25 mm in size. Although tracheal diverticula are connected to the airways by definition, the connecting stalk is frequently below the spatial resolution of a CT scan. These diverticula characteristically present as small air bubbles along the right posterolateral wall of the upper trachea (at the level of T1–T3). However, tracheal diverticula may contain fluid, particularly in patients with cystic fibrosis.[8] Depending on the protein content of the fluid,

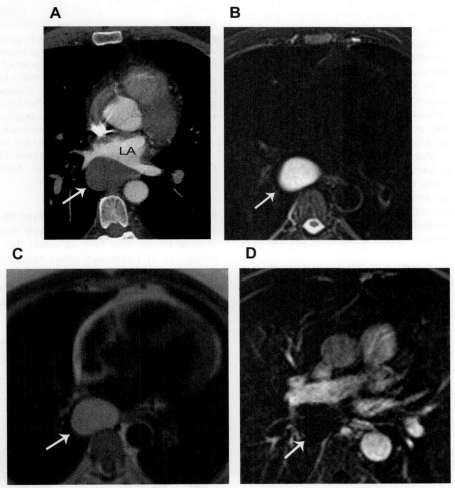

**Fig. 4.** A bronchogenic cyst in a 50-year-old woman with persistent cough. (A) A contrast-enhanced axial CT scan of the chest at the level of the left atrium (LA) demonstrates a homogeneous low attenuation (38 Hounsfield units) mass (arrow) in the visceral mediastinum compressing the left atrium. On CT scan, cysts with hemorrhage or proteinaceous material may demonstrate density similar to soft tissue and can be misinterpreted as solid lesions. (B) An axial T2-weighted MR image demonstrates homogeneous high signal intensity in the lesion (arrow), consistent with a cyst. (C) An axial T1-weighted MR image demonstrates homogeneous high signal intensity relative to muscle (arrow). The high signal intensity on both T1- and T2-weighted images confirms the proteinaceous cyst content. (D) A subtracted fat-suppressed axial T1-weighted MR image after the administration of intravenous gadolinium contrast demonstrates no enhancement of either the lesion or its wall (arrow) and no nodules. MR imaging is the optimal imaging modality for distinguishing cystic from solid lesions, identifying cystic and/or necrotic lesion components, and characterizing cystic lesions as to the presence of septations and mural nodularity.

tracheal diverticula may be misinterpreted as a cyst or a lymph node, which carries implications in the oncologic setting (**Fig. 3**). Although most patients are asymptomatic, some may rarely present with cough owing to pulmonary aspiration or pneumonia, because the diverticula may serve as a reservoir for food residue or secretions.[8,9]

Bronchogenic cysts result from abnormal budding of the primitive foregut, which also gives rise to the tracheobronchial tree, during embryologic development. These benign lesions may arise from any mediastinal compartment, but typically occur in the visceral compartment near the carina or, less commonly, the right paratracheal region. Histologically, bronchogenic cysts are lined by respiratory epithelium and contain a thick mucoid material. Bronchogenic cysts can grow substantially in size without causing symptoms; however, patients may report symptoms when adjacent mediastinal structures are compressed. Bronchogenic cysts typically manifest as well-defined lesions composed of simple fluid. However, when CT attenuation of fluid with a high protein content approaches that of soft tissue, bronchogenic cysts may be misinterpreted as neoplasms. MR imaging adds value by demonstrating the cystic nature with a high signal intensity on T2-weighted images. The signal intensity on T1-weighted images varies depending on the cyst contents (**Fig. 4**).[5]

A Zenker's diverticulum (pharyngeal pouch) is a typical pulsion diverticulum that represents an acquired sac-like posterior outpouching of the hypopharynx proximal to the upper esophageal sphincter through a *locus minoris resistentiae* in the muscular layer (Killian dehiscence). The typical location is at the C5 to C6 level, although extension into the mediastinum may be seen when large.[10,11] Zenker's diverticula usually present in the seventh and eighth decades of life, with a 1.5 times male predominance. Their true prevalence is probably underestimated, because many diverticula remain clinically silent. Although fluoroscopic esophagram is often used to diagnose Zenker's diverticula owing to the dynamic nature of the modality, they may be incidentally detected on a CT scan (**Fig. 5**).

## VASCULAR STRUCTURES

A variety of normal vascular structures may be misinterpreted as pathology in specific circumstances. For example, valves in the azygos and hemiazygos veins may accumulate intravenous contrast and mimic calcified lymph nodes on a CT scan (**Fig. 6**).[12] Flow-related artifacts owing to the mixing of unenhanced and enhanced blood

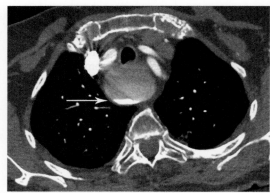

**Fig. 5.** A large Zenker's diverticulum in an 81-year-old woman undergoing CT imaging for pulmonary embolism. A contrast-enhanced axial CT scan of the chest shows a fluid–fluid level (*arrow*) within a large retrotracheal cystic lesion, representing a large Zenker's diverticulum. The layering effect reflects the different attenuation coefficients of various esophageal contents. The content of a Zenker's diverticulum may at times be of high attenuation mimicking intravenous contrast. This should not be mistaken for hemorrhage. When in doubt, a repeat chest CT scan without intravenous contrast may be helpful.

may be mistaken for an intravascular filling defect or thrombus. Obtaining a delayed scan in the venous phase may help to avoid this potential pitfall (**Fig. 7**). Pulmonary artery motion and inspirational flow-related artifacts may simulate a filling defect or dissection. Obtaining a delayed scan in the venous phase or repeating the scan with

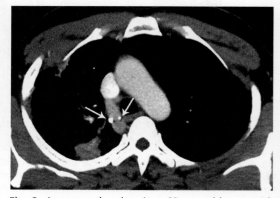

**Fig. 6.** Azygos arch valves in a 68-year-old man with tuberculosis in the right upper lobe. A contrast-enhanced axial CT scan of the chest demonstrates the reflux of intravenous contrast into the azygos vein, lodged within the valves (*arrows*). Knowledge of the typical appearance and location of the azygos arch valves is important in avoiding misinterpretation as calcified lymph nodes, calcified thrombus or a foreign body.

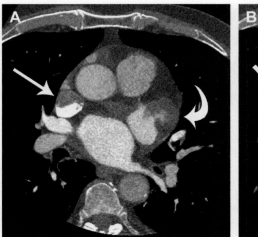
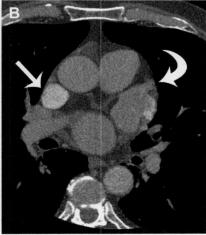

**Fig. 7.** Flow artifact in a 70-year-old man with atrial fibrillation undergoing imaging evaluation for thrombus in the left atrial appendage. (*A*) A contrast-enhanced axial CT scan of the heart in the arterial phase demonstrates a low attenuation focus along the anterior aspect of the superior vena cava (*arrow*). This flow artifact is caused by the mixing and volume averaging of unenhanced blood with contrast-enhanced blood on an arterial phase CT scan. Slow flow within the trabeculated left atrial appendage simulates a thrombus (*curved arrow*). (*B*) A contrast-enhanced axial CT scan of the heart in the delayed phase shows a more homogenous appearance of the superior vena cava (*arrow*) and the left atrial appendage (*curved arrow*). Better mixing of contrast with the blood on delayed phase confirms the absence of thrombus.

ECG gating are solutions to address these issues (**Fig. 8**).[13,14]

## CARDIAC STRUCTURES

Technical advances in CT technology, with faster rotation times and shorter scan durations, lead to better delineation of cardiac structures with less motion artifacts even in the absence of ECG gating. Familiarity with age-related cardiac changes, flow artifacts, and anatomic variations is useful to avoid misinterpretation as cardiac pathology.

Aortic wall motion during the cardiac cycle may result in curvilinear artifacts that characteristically appear in proximity to the aortic root, where the cardiac motion is most prominent. ECG gating increases the diagnostic accuracy and substantially decrease motion artifacts in the aortic root and proximal ascending aorta without increasing radiation exposure (**Fig. 9**).[15–17]

The left atrial appendage (LAA) anatomy is highly variable and complex with multiple prominent trabeculations and thin walls. In patients with atrial fibrillation, slow flow, blood stasis, and thrombus formation often occur and can be challenging to diagnose. Recently, interest in LAA imaging has increased owing to the need to

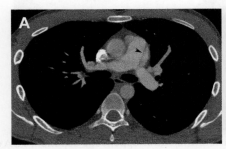
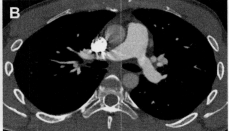

**Fig. 8.** Cardiac motion artifact in a 48-year-old man undergoing imaging after a traumatic injury. (*A*) A contrast-enhanced axial non–ECG-gated CT scan at the level of the pulmonary trunk demonstrates a linear low attenuation band (*arrowhead*) along the long axis of the pulmonary trunk suspicious for pulmonary artery dissection. (*B*) A contrast-enhanced axial ECG-gated CT scan performed the following day demonstrates a normal appearance of the pulmonary trunk. ECG gating is useful in resolving cardiac motion artifact.

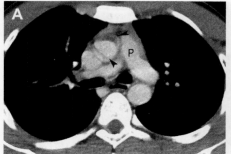
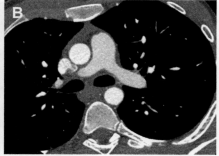

**Fig. 9.** Cardiac motion artifact in a 20-year-old man imaged after a motor vehicle collision. (*A*) A contrast-enhanced axial non–ECG-gated CT scan at the level of the pulmonary trunk (P) demonstrates motion artifact (*arrowheads*) in the ascending aorta mimicking aortic injury. (*B*) A contrast-enhanced axial ECG-gated CT scan subsequently performed demonstrates a normal appearance of the ascending aorta. Awareness of the potential pitfall of cardiac motion artifact on the appearance of cardiovascular structures on non-ECG studies and the need to perform ECG gating when appropriate is important.

make clinical decisions regarding antithrombotic treatment: cardioversion, pulmonary vein ablation and LAA occluder insertion. The accurate detection of an LAA thrombus is important because this entity is the main cause of stroke in nonvalvular atrial fibrillation. Documenting LAA thrombus is crucial in obviating the need for further LAA imaging before cardioversion LAA occlusion or pulmonary vein ablation. The approach to the evaluation of the LAA includes delayed imaging with or without ECG gating, prone positioning, and dual energy or dual source imaging. Delayed

LAA imaging shows the value of sensitivity, specificity, positive predictive value, and negative predictive value of 100%, 99%, 92%, and 100%, respectively, in the detection of thrombus (**Fig. 10**).[18,19]

Congenital left ventricular clefts, diverticula, and aneurysms are usually asymptomatic and discovered incidentally during cross-sectional imaging evaluation. Myocardial crypts or clefts are slit-like invaginations within the left ventricular myocardium, observed mostly between the insertion points between the left and right

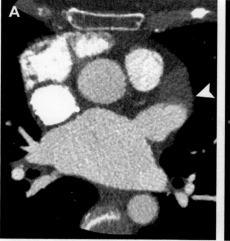
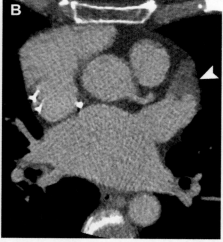

**Fig. 10.** A 68-year-old man undergoing imaging evaluation before left atrial appendage occlusion. (*A*) A contrast-enhanced axial ECG-gated CT scan in the arterial phase demonstrates an apparent filling defect in the nondependent portion of the LAA (*arrowhead*), raising the question of thrombus. This appearance is commonly seen in early phase imaging before the unenhanced blood and contrast enhanced blood have had a chance to mix homogeneously. (*B*) A contrast-enhanced axial ECG-gated CT scan in the venous phase (40-second delay) demonstrates that the LAA filling defect (*arrowhead*) persists confirming the diagnosis of thrombus.

ventricles. Crypts are defined as blood-filled in-vaginations penetrating more than 50% of the myocardial thickness. As CT technological advances lead to greater temporal and spatial resolution, such cardiac findings are visualized more frequently. Myocardial crypts have been reported in normal subjects, hypertrophic cardiomyopathy, aortic stenosis, and hypertension with a reported prevalence of 4% to 9%. Awareness of this entity is essential to avoid misinterpretation and to correlate with relevant underlying clinical conditions (Fig. 11).[18,20,21]

## FAT-CONTAINING STRUCTURES

Fat necrosis abutting the heart, also known as pericardial, epipericardial, or mediastinal fat necrosis, is an uncommon, benign condition of unclear etiology. It is typically located in the cardiophrenic angle, more often on the left. A CT scan usually demonstrates a well-circumscribed round or ovoid mass-like lesion with soft tissue or fat attenuation and adjacent inflammatory changes. On FDG PET/CT scanning, fat necrosis may show increased FDG uptake if imaged during the inflammatory phase. Two clinical scenarios highlight the importance in recognizing this entity. In the symptomatic patient, the detection of fat necrosis as a cause of chest pain aids in avoiding unnecessary additional investigation or invasive procedures. In the asymptomatic patient, awareness of this benign entity is important to avoid misinterpretation as malignancy or lymphadenopathy. When first reported in the literature, patients with fat necrosis had undergone surgical exploration and resection of these lesions. Because epicardial fat necrosis is benign and self-limiting, the current treatment is conservative, with anti-inflammatory agents, and resolution of symptoms

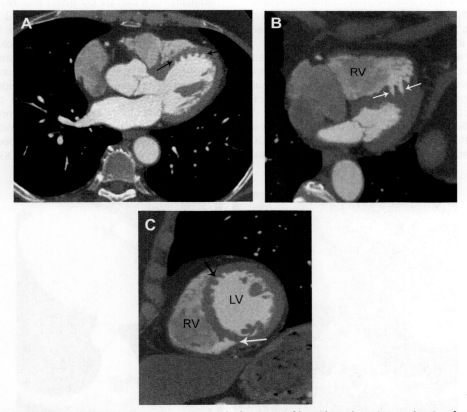

**Fig. 11.** Myocardial crypts in a 65-year-old woman with shortness of breath undergoing evaluation for a pulmonary embolism. (*A*) A contrast-enhanced axial ECG-gated CT scan demonstrates crypts along the left ventricular wall (*black arrows*). (*B*) A contrast-enhanced axial ECG-gated CT scan shows normal right ventricular (RV) myocardial trabeculations (*white arrows*) in the interventricular septum. (*C*)A contrast-enhanced short axis ECG-gated CT scan demonstrates true crypts (*black arrow*) in the left ventricular septum and normal anatomy of the RV wall trabeculations (*white arrow*). In the normal heart, the RV wall is trabeculated, whereas the left ventricular wall is usually smooth.

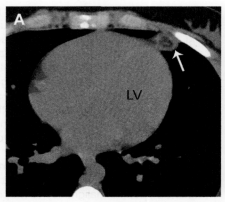
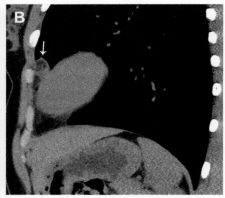

**Fig. 12.** Pericardial and epipericardial fat necrosis in a 20-year-old woman who presented to the emergency department with acute chest pain. (*A*) An unenhanced axial CT scan of the chest demonstrates an oval mass (*arrow*) abutting the left ventricle (LV). There is a soft tissue ring surrounding a fat-containing center and associated mild stranding of the adjacent mediastinal fat. These imaging findings are characteristic of pericardial and epipericardial fat necrosis. (*B*) An unenhanced sagittal reformation demonstrates the oval mass (*arrow*) with stranding of the adjacent mediastinal fat.

within 3 to 4 days after treatment initiation. Knowledge of this entity is important to obtain a correct diagnosis and avoid unnecessary surgical interventions (**Fig. 12**).[22,23]

Brown adipose tissue or fat plays an important role in cold-induced and diet-induced thermogenesis. Brown fat has glucose transporters and can show physiologic FDG uptake, more commonly seen in cold weather and younger individuals. It is typically seen in the supraclavicular regions in a symmetric and elongated distribution on a FDG PET/CT scan. However, when encountered in the

mediastinum, it can be confused with lymphadenopathy on staging or on follow-up FDG PET/CT imaging. Hypermetabolic brown fat in the mediastinum has been reported in 1.8% of oncologic patients, with locations in the paratracheal, paraesophageal, prevascular, and pericardial regions; interatrial septum; and azygoesophageal recess.[24] Knowledge of this potential pitfall is imperative to avoid misinterpretation as nodal disease and lead to errors in the staging and follow-up of oncologic patients. Careful inspection of the CT images to localize the foci of FDG avidity

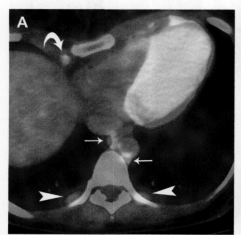
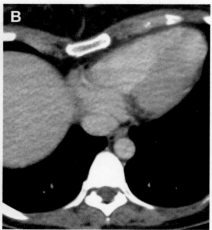

**Fig. 13.** Brown adipose tissue in a 34-year-old woman undergoing follow-up imaging related to melanoma. (*A*) A fused axial FDG PET/CT scan shows foci of increased FDG uptake in the prevascular mediastinum (*curved arrow*), adjacent to the azygous and hemiazygous veins (*arrows*), and in the bilateral paraspinal regions (*arrowheads*). (*B*) A contrast-enhanced axial CT scan of the chest localizes these foci of increased FDG uptake to areas of fat. No lymph nodes were identified in these regions. Deposits of brown adipose tissue can show increased FDG uptake on PET/CT scans owing to cold stimulus.

to areas of fat aids in accurate interpretation (Fig. 13).

## SUMMARY

Potential pitfalls that may be encountered in imaging of the mediastinum include normal structures and variants, various artifacts, and benign lesions that may mimic malignant neoplasms, and may involve cystic, vascular, cardiac, and fat-containing anatomic regions. Familiarity with the variety of potential pitfalls is important to avoid misinterpretation, which may alter patient management and lead to unnecessary investigation and/or procedures.

## CLINICS CARE POINTS

- Advances in multidetector CT technology allow for better delineation of mediastinal structures but also results in the routine visualization of normal anatomic structures and anatomic variants which can be confused with pathology, as well as benign lesions that may mimic malignant neoplasms.
- If a mediastinal mass is suspected to be cystic, MR imaging adds value by demonstrating its fluid content and is helpful to differentiate benign from malignant disease.
- In the symptomatic patient, imaging detection of fat necrosis as a cause of chest pain aids in avoiding unnecessary additional investigation or invasive procedures.

## DISCLOSURE

Nothing to disclose for all authors.

## REFERENCES

1. Tomiyama N, Honda O, Tsubamoto M, et al. Anterior mediastinal tumors: diagnostic accuracy of CT and MRI. Eur J Radiol 2009;69(2):280–8.
2. Shroff GS, Viswanathan C, Godoy MC, et al. Pitfalls in oncologic imaging: pericardial recesses mimicking adenopathy. Semin Roentgenol 2015;50(3):235–40.
3. Roden AC, Fang W, Shen Y, et al. Distribution of mediastinal lesions across multi-institutional, international, radiology databases. J Thorac Oncol 2020;15(4):568–79.
4. Jeung MY, Gasser B, Gangi A, et al. Imaging of cystic masses of the mediastinum. Radiographics 2002;22 Spec No:S79–93.
5. Takeda S, Miyoshi S, Minami M, et al. Clinical spectrum of mediastinal cysts. Chest 2003;124(1):125–32.
6. Ackman JB, Verzosa S, Kovach AE, et al. High rate of unnecessary thymectomy and its cause. Can computed tomography distinguish thymoma, lymphoma, thymic hyperplasia, and thymic cysts? Eur J Radiol 2015;84(3):524–33.
7. Hammer MM, Barile M, Bryson W, et al. Errors in interpretation of magnetic resonance imaging for thymic lesions. J Thorac Imaging 2019;34(6):351–5.
8. Gayer G. Tracheal diverticula. Semin Ultrasound CT MR 2016;37(3):190–5.
9. Gayer G, Sarouk I, Kanaany N, et al. Tracheal diverticula in cystic fibrosis-A potentially important under-reported finding on chest CT. J Cyst Fibros 2016; 15(4):503–9.
10. Bizzotto A, Iacopini F, Landi R, et al. Zenker's diverticulum: exploring treatment options. Acta Otorhinolaryngol Ital 2013;33(4):219–29.
11. Siddiq MA, Sood S, Strachan D. Pharyngeal pouch (Zenker's diverticulum). Postgrad Med J 2001; 77(910):506–11.
12. Yeh BM, Coakley FV, Sanchez HC, et al. Azygos arch valves: prevalence and appearance at contrast-enhanced CT. Radiology 2004;230(1):111–5.
13. Ardley ND, Lau KK, Buchan K, et al. Effects of electrocardiogram gating on CT pulmonary angiography image quality. J Med Imaging Radiat Oncol 2014; 58(3):303–11.
14. Gosselin MV, Rassner UA, Thieszen SL, et al. Contrast dynamics during CT pulmonary angiogram: analysis of an inspiration associated artifact. J Thorac Imaging 2004;19(1):1–7.
15. Bolen MA, Popovic ZB, Tandon N, et al. Image quality, contrast enhancement, and radiation dose of ECG-triggered high-pitch CT versus non-ECG-triggered standard-pitch CT of the thoracoabdominal aorta. AJR Am J Roentgenol 2012;198(4):931–8.
16. Schernthaner RE, Stadler A, Beitzke D, et al. Dose modulated retrospective ECG-gated versus non-gated 64-row CT angiography of the aorta at the same radiation dose: comparison of motion artifacts, diagnostic confidence and signal-to-noise-ratios. Eur J Radiol 2012;81(4):e585–90.
17. Stein E, Mueller GC, Sundaram B. Thoracic aorta (multidetector computed tomography and magnetic resonance evaluation). Radiol Clin North Am 2014; 52(1):195–217.
18. Budoff MJ, Shittu A, Hacioglu Y, et al. Comparison of transesophageal echocardiography versus computed tomography for detection of left atrial appendage filling defect (thrombus). Am J Cardiol 2014;113(1):173–7.
19. Romero J, Husain SA, Kelesidis I, et al. Detection of left atrial appendage thrombus by cardiac computed tomography in patients with atrial fibrillation: a meta-analysis. Circ Cardiovasc Imaging 2013;6(2):185–94.
20. Maron MS, Rowin EJ, Lin D, et al. Prevalence and clinical profile of myocardial crypts in hypertrophic cardiomyopathy. Circ Cardiovasc Imaging 2012; 5(4):441–7.
21. Petryka J, Baksi AJ, Prasad SK, et al. Prevalence of inferobasal myocardial crypts among

patients referred for cardiovascular magnetic resonance. Circ Cardiovasc Imaging 2014;7(2): 259–64.

22. Gayer G. Mediastinal (Epipericardial) fat necrosis: an overlooked and little known cause of acute chest pain mimicking acute coronary syndrome. Semin Ultrasound CT MR 2017;38(6):629–33.

23. Giassi KS, Costa AN, Bachion GH, et al. Epipericardial fat necrosis: who should be a candidate? AJR Am J Roentgenol 2016;207(4):773–7.

24. Truong MT, Erasmus JJ, Munden RF, et al. Focal FDG uptake in mediastinal brown fat mimicking malignancy: a potential pitfall resolved on PET/CT. AJR Am J Roentgenol 2004;183(4):1127–32.

# Image-Guided Biopsies and Interventions of Mediastinal Lesions

Soheil Kooraki, MD[a], Fereidoun Abtin, MD[b],*

## KEYWORDS

- Mediastinal biopsy • Tissue sampling • Mediastinal tumor • Mediastinal ablation • Cryoablation

## KEY POINTS

- For mediastinal biopsies, image guidance is necessary for targeting the lesion and developing an overall plan. Although computed tomography is the most common imaging modality used for this purpose, ultrasound may be used in some scenarios.
- Mediastinal biopsy using a coaxial needle and gun has gained acceptance over fine-needle aspiration due to increased accuracy, particularly for lymphoma.
- To avoid complications and ensure patient safety, biopsy needles should not be targeted toward pulsating organs or vascular structures.
- Mediastinal ablation procedures for limited metastasis and recurrent tumor after initial surgical resection or radiation therapy are being performed more frequently.
- Cryoablation for mediastinal neoplasms is well tolerated by patients, although the heat sink can lead to incomplete ablation and local recurrence.

## INTRODUCTION

Management of mediastinal masses requires accurate diagnosis to develop appropriate treatment strategies. Image-guided transthoracic biopsy of mediastinal lesions is a minimally invasive and relatively safe procedure that can be used to obtain histologic samples under local anesthesia and conscious sedation, tailor the treatment plans, and potentially obviate more invasive diagnostic procedures. Not all mediastinal masses require biopsy, as certain lesions demonstrate characteristic imaging features that enable diagnosis. Examples of such entities that can be solely diagnosed on clinical and imaging characteristics are retrosternal goiter and asymptomatic visceral compartment cystic lesions such as bronchogenic cyst or esophageal duplication cyst.[1] In addition, in certain clinical conditions, transthoracic needle biopsy of a mediastinal lesion is contraindicated, including uncontrollable cough, bleeding diathesis (international normalized ratio [INR]>1.4; platelet count <50000/mL; increased prothrombin time with INR>1.5 or partial thromboplastin time >1.5 times greater than the normal range), bullous emphysema, and moderate-to-severe pulmonary hypertension. In addition, when there is a characteristic hydatid cyst or a vascular lesion on computed tomography (CT), biopsy should be avoided.[2–4]

Image-guided transthoracic needle biopsy is regarded as the reliable, cost-effective, and standard method of choice for obtaining specimens from mediastinal lesions. Biopsy planning can be performed via CT, magnetic resonance (MR)

[a] Department of Nuclear Medicine, University of California Los Angeles (UCLA), 11301 Wilshire Boulevard, Los Angeles, CA 90073, USA; [b] Thoracic and Interventional Section, Department of Radiological Sciences, David Geffen School of Medicine at UCLA, 757 Westwood Plaza, Suite 1621, Los Angeles, CA 90095, USA
* Corresponding author. Santa Monica Out-Patient Center, 1245 16th Street, Suite # 100, Santa Monica, CA 90404.
E-mail address: fabtin@mednet.ucla.edu

Radiol Clin N Am 59 (2021) 291–303
https://doi.org/10.1016/j.rcl.2020.11.009
0033-8389/21/© 2020 Elsevier Inc. All rights reserved.

imaging or ultrasound. Each of these methods has its inherent advantages and disadvantages. Percutaneous image-guided sampling is performed by fine-needle aspiration or core needle biopsy. The choice of technique depends on the lesion characteristics, location, patient comorbidities, and the experience of the operating physician.

This article reviews the various image-guided strategies for biopsy of mediastinal lesions with focus on the diagnostic yield, clinical relevance, technical aspects of biopsy performance, and possible complications. The role of mediastinal ablation for treating conditions such as limited mediastinal metastasis and recurrent thymoma and malignant pleural mesothelioma will also be described. Finally, the use of image guidance for draining mediastinal collections and benign cystic lesions is briefly discussed.

## IMAGING MODALITIES AND CLINICAL RELEVANCE

Image-guided mediastinal biopsy can be performed using different modalities including CT, MR imaging, and ultrasound, with CT remaining, which is used most frequently. The diagnostic yield is defined as the proportion of the diagnostic results achieved by image-guided biopsy, whereas diagnostic accuracy is the proportion of the correct diagnoses relative to the final diagnosis of the lesion. Overall, lymphoma and thymoma are the most common mediastinal mass lesions diagnosed with image-guided biopsy.

Tissue diagnosis is an essential step for management of prevascular mediastinal lesions, except in those with typical imaging features of a cyst. Image-guided biopsy is the least invasive initial method to obtain tissue, as it can obviate more invasive procedures such as mediastinoscopy and anterior mediastinotomy. The sensitivity of needle biopsy in diagnosing prevascular mediastinal lesions depends on tumor type. Most of the nondiagnostic mediastinal biopsies are later diagnosed as lymphoma. The diagnostic yield of percutaneous biopsy for mediastinal lymphoma varies and is based on the pathologic subtype of lymphoma. Fine-needle aspiration has low diagnostic yield for lymphoma, whereas core needle biopsy increases the diagnostic accuracy, in particular, for Hodgkin lymphoma.[5]

### Computed Tomography

CT is the most commonly used modality for localization of mediastinal lesions and documentation of biopsy needle track.[6] A meta-analysis of 1345 CT-guided core needle biopsies of mediastinal masses from 18 studies found pooled diagnostic yield of 92% with 94% diagnostic accuracy. They showed that diagnostic yield and accuracy were significantly higher in studies with 3 or higher sampled cores.[7] CT scan allows for accurate targeting and assesses for complications during and immediately after biopsy, for example, pneumothorax or pleural effusion, which can be missed with ultrasound.

### MR Imaging

MR imaging may have some advantages over CT, including its superior soft tissue resolution, real-time multiplanar imaging capabilities, excellent delineation of the vascular structures, and lack of ionizing radiation. It is also the preferred modality to assess the paravertebral lesions with possible neural origin. MR imaging, however, is limited by higher costs, longer procedure time, motion artifact, and paramagnetic artifact from usual biopsy needles, which can limit visualization of small lesions or the needle trajectory path in some patients. Garnon and colleagues were the first to describe the use of MR-targeted biopsy of mediastinal lesions in 16 individuals using wide-bore high-filed scanner. They reported a technical success and accuracy of 100% and 87.5%, respectively, with a mean procedure duration of 42 minutes, without any immediate complications.[8]

### Ultrasound

Certain mediastinal lesions may be accessible through ultrasound guidance. The technique is practical when the mediastinal lesions are adequately imaged by ultrasound, including those located in the high prevascular mediastinum or those that are adjacent to or protrude through the chest wall. Ultrasound is cost-effective, time saving, and feasible for sampling of mediastinal lesions with diagnostic yield of 80% to 100%.[9–12] Advantages of ultrasound are continuous real-time needle and target visualization, the ability for oblique needle placement, needle slope manipulation or changing the patient's position during procedure, and the possibility to perform the targeted biopsy at the bedside of critically ill patients. These features are difficult or impossible to perform under CT guidance. The additional use of color Doppler ultrasound can help avoid the vascular structures during procedure.[13] The main limitation of ultrasound is the limited acoustic window. In the largest series of ultrasound-guided biopsies of mediastinal lesions, Petkov and colleagues[12] evaluated the efficacy of using ultrasound guidance for sampling mediastinal masses larger than 15 mm in 566 patients. The target lesion was visible on ultrasound in 54.4% (91.9% in prevascular, 0.6% in visceral, and 7.5% in paravertebral mediastinum) of the study cohort, in whom ultrasound-guided core needle biopsy was performed. In the individuals with nonvisible lesions on ultrasound, CT-guided transthoracic core needle biopsy was performed. The diagnostic yield of ultrasound-guided biopsy was 96%, comparable with 90% diagnostic accuracy in CT-guided biopsy.

The application of contrast-enhanced ultrasound can increase the diagnostic yield and diagnostic accuracy of biopsy compared with conventional ultrasound guidance. Contrast-enhanced ultrasound allows detection of necrotic and nonviable areas within the mass to be precluded from sampling.[14,15]

## TECHNICAL CONSIDERATIONS
### Needle Selection

Several types of needles with different caliber can be used for sampling mediastinal lesions. Needle selection depends on the presumptive diagnosis, size of the lesion, lesion depth from skin, proximity of the vital structures to the biopsy path, and the operating radiologist experience. Cutting-bore or Tru-Cut guns, ranging from 14 to 20 gauge in caliber, can be used to obtain specimen for histologic evaluation and are usually introduced through a coaxial needle. The most common size combination is the 19-gauge coaxial needle and 20-gauge gun. Aspiration needles, ranging from 20 to 23 gauge in caliber are used for cytologic evaluation. Adequate tissue target sampling and diagnostic accuracy are more achievable using core needle biopsy than fine-needle aspiration.[16] Fine-needle aspiration has high sensitivity for obtaining tissue specimens from cystic masses or malignant metastatic lesions; however, it has a relatively low diagnostic yield for the diagnosis of lymphoma. A combination of fine-needle and multiple (ie, 3–5) core needle biopsies has higher diagnostic performance for this purpose. Overall, fine-needle aspiration was the preferred strategy in lesions that are adjacent to vital structures (such as the great vessels), in transpulmonary approach for biopsy, and specifically when a metastatic disease is the first clinical impression.[16] Currently, the most common biopsy technique uses the coaxial system, which is preferred by most radiologists. The guide coaxial needle is placed in a position near or in the target lesion and then a biopsy gun is advanced through the coaxial system to obtain the specimen. Coaxial systems help reduce the number of passes and the possibility of iatrogenic injury to the vital structures. Larger caliber guns can provide much better tissue samples for genetic analysis and hence improve genomic sequencing in particular for lymphoma. In circumstances where tissue is accessible and size of tumor is larger than 1.5 cm, 17-/18-gauge coaxial/gun systems are preferred.[17]

### Biopsy Procedure

Image-guided mediastinal biopsy is routinely performed under conscious sedation by using midazolam and/or fentanyl citrate. In noncooperative patients and in pediatric patients, deep sedation or general anesthesia is usually necessary. Local anesthetics (eg, 5–10 mL 1% solution of Lidocaine) are administered before the procedure. Patients may be placed in the supine, prone, or lateral decubitus position based on the selected biopsy approach and the anatomic location of the target lesion. Simple positioning of the patient in the oblique decubitus can allow for mediastinal shift and the mass to move into an accessible needle trajectory approach in order to avoid traversing lung. Before beginning the procedure, the lesion is reassessed on previously acquired cross-sectional images or ultrasound. When prior fluorodeoxyglucose (FDG) PET/CT is available, the most FDG-avid portions of the mediastinal mass lesion are targeted. Repeat imaging examination may be necessary based on the individual case. When planning the path for the needle, it is important to choose a course that allows for the needle to be tangential to the mediastinal vessels in order to avoid targeting the needle toward pulsating organs or vascular structures.

For CT-guided biopsy, unenhanced CT with 3 mm slices is generally adequate to plan the procedure. In select high-risk cases, however, the use of intravenous contrast material could help delineate vascular structures, especially those that may be engulfed by tumor, in the needle trajectory. The optimal CT section is then marked on the skin with the axial laser localizer of the scanner. Radiopaque markers are positioned along the laser light beam, and the scan is repeated to localize the exact point of entry (Fig. 1A). A radiopaque marker is then replaced with a skin mark using an indelible pen. A repeat localizer CT is required in each step of needle advancement to ensure the safety of needle trajectory and readjust the biopsy needle when necessary (Fig. 1B). When the mediastinal fat contact with the biopsy needle is not satisfactory to ensure a safe needle trajectory, injection of physiologic saline or dilute contrast medium into the mediastinum can create a safe

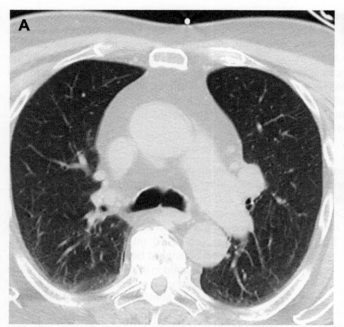
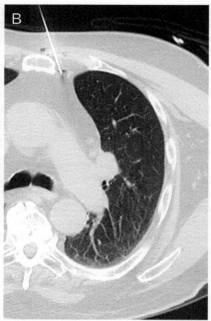

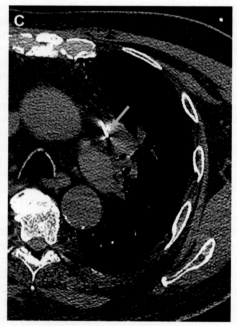

**Fig. 1.** CT-guided biopsy of left prevascular mediastinal mass. (*A*) A radiopaque marker is used on the skin to plan the trajectory. (*B*) The coaxial needle is incrementally advanced into the mediastinum. Using a parasternal approach, the needle is placed between the internal mammary vessels and sternum. Lidocaine can be used to displace the vessels away from the needle trajectory. (*C*) The needle is incrementally advanced until it is located within the lesion of interest (*arrow*).

extrapleural path for performing the biopsy[18] (**Fig. 1**).

For ultrasound-guided mediastinal biopsy procedures, a sector (2.0–2.5 MHz), convex (3.5–5–7.5 MHz), or linear (5–7.5–12.0 MHz) array transducer may be used by the operating radiologist based on the depth of the target lesion from skin and the available acoustic window. The gray scale B-mode imaging is used to direct the needle toward the target lesion, frequently accompanied by color doppler imaging to avoid the mediastinal vessels. In addition, a twinkling sign on color doppler ultrasound allows visualization of the biopsy needle. Needles may be introduced using a free-hand technique or a stretcher guide attached to the transducer. The free-hand technique allows manual movement of the needle into the target lesion under direct visualization.

When the radiologist will be acquiring specimens, it is important to be familiar with the biopsy system, particularly the loading of the gun and the extent of the "throw" beyond the coaxial needle. Injury by extension of the gun into vital structures is unacceptable. The number of samples obtained depends on the suspected disease and the radiologist's confidence. Typically, 2 to 5 cores are obtained per target lesion.

Iatrogenic pneumothorax can be used for mediastinal access without traversing a diseased lung. This approach adds extra time to the procedure but provides a much quicker recovery (**Fig. 2**).

Following the biopsy, patients may be observed on the scanner for 5 to 10 minutes to confirm the absence of bleeding before moving the patient to an observation unit. Patients are generally observed for at least 2 hours after the procedure to ensure hemodynamic stability and to monitor respiratory status. Imaging with chest radiographs or CT fluoroscopy is performed immediately after the procedure and 2 hours after the biopsy in patients in whom the pleura was punctured or when there has been respiratory distress.

## Interventional Approaches

Mediastinal lesions can be accessed through parasternal, transsternal, suprasternal, paravertebral, subxiphoid, transpleural, and transpulmonary approaches. A transthyroid approach can also be attempted to access a retrotracheal target lesion. Transgression of the brachiocephalic vein using a small-caliber fine-needle aspiration needle is a safe and applicable method to obtain samples from target lesions through suprasternal, substernal, and parasternal approaches.

### Parasternal

The parasternal route is the most common approach for sampling prevascular and visceral mediastinal lesions, specifically those that are located in the prevascular, pretracheal, paratracheal, and aorticopulmonary window stations. The technique is feasible under CT or ultrasound guidance. The biopsy needle is inserted lateral to the sternum, and the lesion is reached through the parasternal muscles and mediastinal fat. It is important to identify the internal thoracic arteries and veins to prevent vascular injury during the procedure.[19] The internal thoracic vessels can be identified within 2.5 cm of the either side of the sternum. The needle is placed either medial or lateral to the internal thoracic vessels that can be displaced by injecting saline with or without lidocaine (see **Fig. 1**B). In an ultrasound-guided parasternal approach, a small footprint probe is

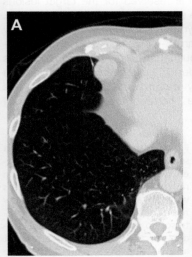 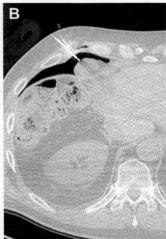 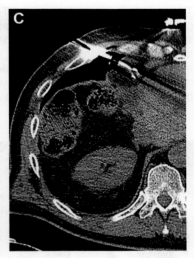

**Fig. 2.** CT-guided biopsy of endometrial carcinoma metastasis. (*A*) Unenhanced axial CT demonstrates the metastasis in the right cardiophrenic angle of the right prevascular mediastinum. (*B*) A coaxial needle was used to induce a small pneumothorax (*arrow*) followed by introduction of a second needle for biopsy and histopathological evaluation. (*C*) At the same visit, following the confirmation of metastasis, the lesion was treated with cryoablation. Two probes are present in the lesion, and a low-density cryozone ("iceball") is seen surrounding the tumor.

required considering the limited acoustic window resulting from anterior curvature of the ribs and costal cartilages (**Fig. 3**).

### Transsternal

This approach is reserved for prevascular mediastinal lesions, which are not readily accessible visceral and paravertebral mediastinal compartment lesions.[20] Mediastinal lesions can be accessed by this method without traversing pulmonary parenchyma or the risk of injury to internal thoracic vessels. The procedure, however, carries a small risk of injury to major vessels in the prevascular mediastinum. A coaxial bone biopsy system with an eccentric drill is used in this method. The procedure is performed under local anesthesia, and the anesthetic agent is administered to coat the anterior and posterior sternal periosteum (**Fig. 4**). Injection of the anesthetic agent before puncturing the posterior cortex of sternum can decrease possible patient discomfort.[20–22] The technique, however, has several limitations. It is not feasible in patients with previous sternotomy. In addition, the needle trajectory cannot be manipulated after sternal insertion. Further movement of arms and thorax cavity should be minimized after needle insertion, as it might alter the anatomy of the mediastinal mass. The amount of contact between sternum and mediastinum might change during biopsy, which can potentially cause pleural damage.

### Suprasternal

This approach is practical under CT or ultrasound guidance for sampling high mediastinal lesions, specifically those that are located in the prevascular, pretracheal, right paratracheal, or aorticopulmonary window stations. The needle needs to be directed caudally while patient is lying in the supine position with a hyperextended neck.[10,23]

### Paravertebral

This route is used for sampling paravertebral mediastinal and subcarinal lesions.[24–26] The patient may be placed in the prone, prone oblique, or lateral decubitus position, and the needle is introduced typically from right paravertebral space, between the endothoracic fascia and the parietal pleura to access the target lesion. When the access route is not wide enough, saline or dilute contrast material can be used for widening the extrapleural paravertebral space and displacing the mediastinal structures out of the needle path (**Fig. 5**). This approach can potentially cause injury to esophagus, azygos vein, vagus nerve, and intercostal vessels and nerves.[25]

### Subxiphoid

A subxiphoid approach is used for drainage of pericardial effusions and sampling pericardial masses.[27] In this approach, the needle is placed below the xiphoid process and is angled cranially under CT or ultrasound guidance.

### Transpleural

This approach is performed under CT guidance and requires the presence of a large pleural effusion or pneumothorax as a window. The patient position is flexible, and, therefore, this path might be beneficial for patients who have dyspnea and difficulty lying supine or in the prone positions.[24]

### Transpulmonary

This approach is reserved for the target lesions that cannot be safely accessed with other routes. Mediastinal lymph nodes can be efficiently sampled with an 18-gauge core coaxial needle using the transpulmonary route. The procedure is performed under CT guidance with penetration of the pulmonary parenchyma and pleural layers and therefore carries the highest risk of

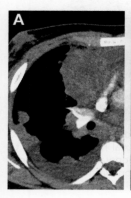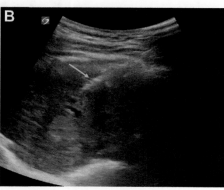

**Fig. 3.** Ultrasound-guided biopsy of a seminoma metastasis. (*A*) Contrast-enhanced axial CT demonstrates the right prevascular mediastinal mass with an adequate acoustic window for ultrasound-guided biopsy. (*B*) Ultrasound image shows a coaxial needle in the mass with a bright acoustic shadow (*arrow*). The edge of the sternum and intercostal muscles are clearly delineated with ultrasound.

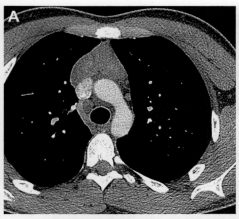
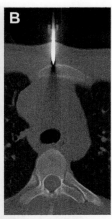

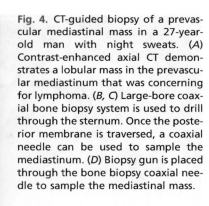

Fig. 4. CT-guided biopsy of a prevascular mediastinal mass in a 27-year-old man with night sweats. (*A*) Contrast-enhanced axial CT demonstrates a lobular mass in the prevascular mediastinum that was concerning for lymphoma. (*B, C*) Large-bore coaxial bone biopsy system is used to drill through the sternum. Once the posterior membrane is traversed, a coaxial needle can be used to sample the mediastinum. (*D*) Biopsy gun is placed through the bone biopsy coaxial needle to sample the mediastinal mass.

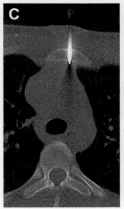
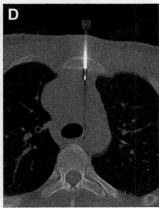

pneumothorax and alveolar hemorrhage, compared with other routes[24,28,29] (**Fig. 6**).

## MEDIASTINAL ABLATIONS

Over the past several years, ablation modalities have improved to allow for treatment of an ever-expanding list of indications and placement of needles into the mediastinum for performing the procedures. Radiofrequency ablation was the initial ablation modality used in the mediastinum, with a series performed on mediastinal lymph nodes[30] demonstrating local control of up to 75% at 1 year for lymph nodes below 2 cm. However, the control was poor for lymph nodes larger than 2 cm.

Another more common indication for mediastinal ablation is local control of tumor following surgical resection or radiation therapy. Cryoablation has been used to provide local control of disease in patients with recurrent malignant pleural mesothelioma with many of the recurrences in the prevascular and paravertebral mediastinum. These recurrences were treated with cryoablation with a local control rate of 100% of cases at 30 days,

92.5% at 6 months, 90.8% at 1 year, 87.3% at 2 years, and 73.7% at 3 years[31] (**Fig. 7**). Another cohort that benefited from ablation was patients with thymoma who had undergone surgical resection with local recurrence and distant drop metastasis.[32] Cryoablation of these recurrent tumors provided local control of up to 90%. The recurrences after ablation were seen next to the thoracic aorta, which did not allow for complete ablation due to heat sink effect from the aorta.

Another indication for mediastinal ablation is the possible abscopal effect it may have during ongoing treatment with immunotherapy. Cryoablation is known to release tumor antigens that can induce an immune response against distant tumor cells; however, this immune response may not be large enough, and combining cryoablation with immune modulators has been shown to have a more symbiotic and robust response (**Fig. 8**).

## OTHER IMAGE-GUIDED INTERVENTIONS

Percutaneous image-guided drainage can be used for treatment of mediastinal abscesses,

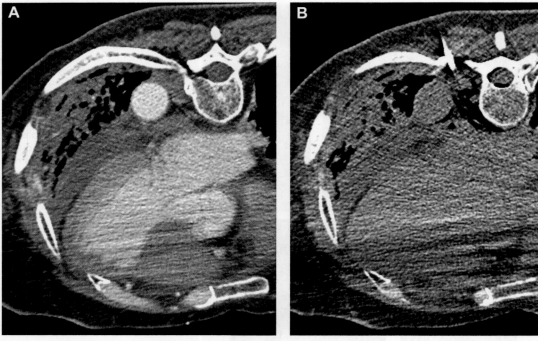

**Fig. 5.** CT-guided biopsy of a paravertebral mediastinal mass in a patient with prior thymoma. (*A*) Contrast-enhanced axial CT demonstrates a mass in the paravertebral mediastinum insinuating itself between the aorta and the spine. (*B*) A paravertebral approach is used to biopsy the lesion that was confirmed as recurrence.

which result from esophageal perforation, infectious process, or iatrogenic injuries.[33,34] The trocar and Seldinger techniques are the two standard approaches commonly used. The tandem trocar technique is a single-step procedure in which a localizing needle is first placed into the mediastinal collection followed by enlargement of a skin incision using a metal forceps and, finally, pushing a drainage catheter parallel (tandem) to the localizing needle. This technique is typically feasible for drainage of large and superficial collections. In the Seldinger technique, a 17- to 19-gauge needle is placed into the mediastinal collection and a fluid sample is obtained, followed by the

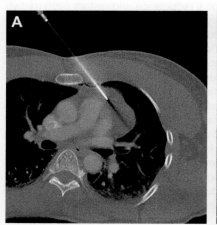
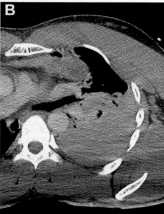
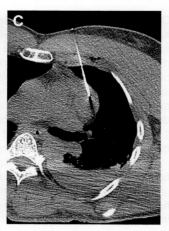

**Fig. 6.** CT-guided biopsy of a prevascular mediastinal mass in a 47-year-old woman. (*A*) Parasternal approach was selected for targeting the mass. (*B*) After obtaining the first sample, the patient complained of excruciating pain. A subsequent CT image demonstrates mediastinal and left pleural hemorrhage. (*C*) A repeat biopsy was performed 3 days later using a transpulmonary approach.

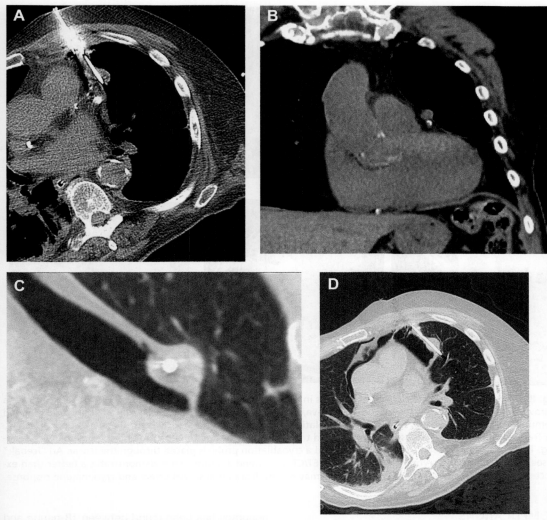

**Fig. 7.** CT-guided biopsy of recurrent mesothelioma. (*A, B*) CT images show that a prevascular mediastinal approach was used to place the cryoablation probe into the recurrent mesothelioma. (*C, D*) Pneumomediastinum was induced to displace the tumor from the left anterior descending coronary artery. The probe was also angulated laterally to increase the gap. Cryoablation was performed without any complications.

advancement of an 8- to 16-French pigtail catheter over a guidewire into the fluid collection. Both techniques require frequent intermittent CT acquisition during the procedure. Once the catheter location is confirmed inside the collection, the catheter is secured to the skin. Complete resolution is reported in 95.6% of the patients, with a mean catheter drainage time of 13.6 days, obviating further surgical intervention.[33] CT-guided drainage is also potentially useful for treatment of postoperative collections including those related to esophageal anastomotic leaks. Typically, surgical intervention is used for tissue debridement and mediastinal drainage in patients with

postoperative anastomotic leak. If a CT-guided procedure is preferred, the drainage catheter needs to be placed close to the anastomotic leakage site to ensure effective drainage.[35]

Bronchogenic cysts may require therapeutic intervention when they produce significant clinical symptoms. Percutaneous transthoracic needle aspiration is an effective method for confirming the diagnosis and draining a suspected bronchogenic cyst. Simple aspiration may cause recurrence due to incomplete obliteration of the cyst lining; therefore, intracystic sclerotherapy with a sclerosant agent such as ethanol or bleomycin may be more efficient.[36,37]

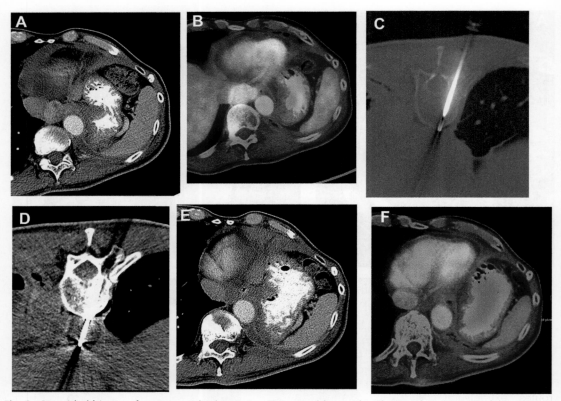

**Fig. 8.** CT-guided biopsy of a paravertebral mass in a 72-year-old man. (*A, B*) CT and FDG PET/CT demonstrate a paravertebral mass between the inferior vena cava, esophagus, and heart. Given the solitary lesion and planned immunotherapy, the plan was to perform cryoablation to take advantage of local control and abscopal effect. (*C, D*) Transvertebral approach was selected to avoid traversing the contralateral pleura and the possibility of seeding. The bone trocar is used to create a tract, and a cryoablation probe is placed through the trocar. An "iceball" is seen surrounding the cryoprobes. (*E, F*) FDG PET/CT performed 3 months later demonstrates a better than expected response to cryoablation, which may or may not be from an abscopal effect and cryoimmune response.

## COMPLICATIONS

Several postprocedural complications have been described in image-guided mediastinal biopsies, including pneumothorax, chest wall hematoma, hemothorax, hemoptysis, and vasovagal syncope.[25] In a meta-analysis of 1345 core needle biopsies of mediastinal lesions, the total complication rate and major complication rates were 13% and 2%, respectively.[7] The figures are significantly lower than the reported complication rate of 38.8% for CT-guided lung biopsy mainly because of the lower rate of pneumothorax.[38] Biopsy of lesions in the visceral mediastinum is associated with a relatively higher risk of postprocedural complications, of which hemorrhage is the most common complication[39] (see **Fig. 6**B). The application of a small-caliber needle (18 gauge or higher) is associated with a significant decrease in the rate of postprocedural complications. Because no significant difference in the diagnostic accuracy has been found between 18-gauge and 20-gauge needles in the meta-analysis by Lee and colleagues,[7] the use of 20-gauge needle for core needle biopsy of mediastinal lesions may be sufficient, with the exception of lymphomas, which may require a greater amount of tissue.

Alveolar hemorrhage and hemoptysis are rare and mainly occur when the pulmonary parenchyma is markedly traversed by the biopsy needle (eg, when a transpulmonary approach is used for sampling the target lesion). Pneumothorax is by far the most common complication of transthoracic mediastinal biopsy. Small self-resolving pneumothoraces occur in 3.8% of CT-guided biopsy of prevascular mediastinal lesions.[5] The transpulmonary approach has the highest risk of pneumothorax. The most significant risk factors for developing pneumothorax in this technique include the distance between the pleura and the target lesion and the number of times in which the visceral pleura is penetrated.[28] Several

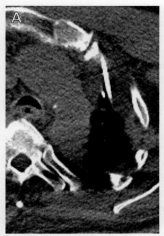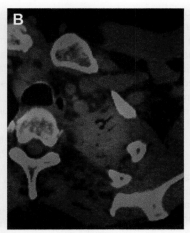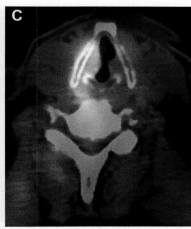

Fig. 9. CT-guided biopsy of recurrent mesothelioma. (A) CT demonstrates cryoablation with the hypodense "iceball" surrounding the needle and encroaching on the aortic arch. This trajectory is the expected location of the path taken by the recurrent laryngeal nerve. (B, C) FDG PET/CT obtained after ablation demonstrates residual ablation zone with no metabolic activity. However, evaluation of the vocal cords shows no activity in the left vocal cord, confirming paralysis due to nerve injury.

strategies may help decrease the rate of pneumothorax,[24] including the use of safer biopsy approaches such as transsternal and suprasternal routes, extrapleural saline injection,[40] manipulating patient position, and a protective "artificial pneumothorax." In the artificial pneumothorax technique,[41] about 200 mL of air is administered into the pleural space to deviate the lung away from the trajectory of the biopsy path and to sample the target lesion through air-containing pleura. After collecting satisfactory samples, the air is aspirated from the pleural space (see Fig. 2). If a pneumothorax develops during the procedure, the pleural air can be aspirated using the introducer needle or a separate needle.[42] An 18- to 20-gauge coaxial needle or small caliber catheter is inserted into the pleural space under real-time CT fluoroscopy and, using an extension tube and a 3-way stopcock, is connected to a 20 to 50 mL syringe. Manual pleural air aspiration by this method obviates use of chest tube placement in roughly 85% of the patients. When a pneumothorax persists, or is recurrent or large, chest tube placement should be considered.

It is stated that ultrasound-guided biopsy has lower complication rates than CT-guided biopsy. For example, Petkov and colleagues[12] reported a complication rate of 2.6% with ultrasound guidance versus 14.6% with CT guidance. The findings need to be interpreted with caution, as CT guidance is chosen for difficult-to-access or sonographically invisible lesions, which are more prone to procedural complications.

Nerve injury is uncommon with biopsies and is more frequent with ablations. The nerves most commonly injured include the recurrent laryngeal nerve, lower trunk of the brachial plexus, and the phrenic nerve. It is essential to plan the ablation with accurate understanding of nerve anatomy and using dissection techniques with fluid or air to avoid injury.[43] However, there are times in which the nerve may need to be sacrificed to obtain complete ablation and cover the tumor margins (Fig. 9).

## FUTURE DIRECTIONS

In the era of precision medicine, patient-specific, evidence-based planning for sampling of mediastinal lesions is of great importance. The use of advanced imaging techniques with combination anatomic and functional information such as PET/CT allows localization of the specific component of the target lesion for more precise biopsy planning. The use of fusion techniques and development of robotic-assisted devices and navigational systems will improve access to target lesions, decrease the procedure time, and increase the accuracy. Several more flexible needles are being developed, which will allow steering the needle from outside of the body to reach to the specific target.

## SUMMARY

Image-guided biopsy is safe and associated with high diagnostic yield and accuracy for histologic evaluation of mediastinal masses. Although CT remains the imaging modality of choice image guidance, ultrasound and MR imaging can be used in certain clinical scenarios. Mediastinal ablation can be performed in select patients with an ever-expanding list of indications and adequate local control rate. Finally, CT-guided drainage is an effective procedure for treatment of mediastinal collections and benign cystic lesions.

## CLINICS CARE POINTS

- Image guided biopsy of mediastinal lesions is safe and provides a high diagnostic yield.
- The choice of imaging modality and the biopsy approach should be decided on a patient-by-patient basis.
- The core needle biopsy has a higher diagnostic yield for the diagnosis of mediastinal lymphoma.
- The coaxial system is the preferred method of sampling mediastinal lesions.
- Cryoablation of recurrent thymoma or malignant pleural mesothelioma has a short-term local control rate of 90-100%.
- Image-guided drainage is a safe and effective procedure for the treatment of mediastinal collections and benign mediastinal cystic lesions.

## DISCLOSURE

The authors have nothing to disclose.

## REFERENCES

1. Tannous HCJ, Yammine MB. Mediastinal masses. In: DJSP E, editor. Clinical algorithm in general surgery. Cham (Switzerland): Springer; 2019. p. 39–41.
2. Westcott JL. Percutaneous transthoracic needle biopsy. Radiology 1988;169(3):593–601.
3. Perlmutt LM, Johnston WW, Dunnick NR. Percutaneous transthoracic needle aspiration: a review. AJR Am J Roentgenol 1989;152(3):451–5.
4. Zafar N, Moinuddin S. Mediastinal needle biopsy. A 15-year experience with 139 cases. Cancer 1995; 76(6):1065–8.
5. Petranovic M, Gilman MD, Muniappan A, et al. Diagnostic yield of CT-guided percutaneous transthoracic needle biopsy for diagnosis of anterior mediastinal masses. AJR Am J Roentgenol 2015; 205(4):774–9.
6. Kulkarni S, Kulkarni A, Roy D, et al. Percutaneous computed tomography-guided core biopsy for the diagnosis of mediastinal masses. Ann Thorac Med 2008;3(1):13–7.
7. Lee HN, Yun SJ, Kim JI, et al. Diagnostic outcome and safety of CT-guided core needle biopsy for

mediastinal masses: a systematic review and meta-analysis. Eur Radiol 2020;30(1):588–99.
8. Garnon J, Ramamurthy N, Caudrelier JJ, et al. MRI-guided percutaneous biopsy of mediastinal masses using a large bore magnet: technical feasibility. Cardiovasc Intervent Radiol 2016;39(5): 761–7.
9. Andersson T, Lindgren PG, Elvin A. Ultrasound guided tumour biopsy in the anterior mediastinum. An alternative to thoracotomy and mediastinoscopy. Acta Radiol 1992;33(5):423–6.
10. Gupta S, Gulati M, Rajwanshi A, et al. Sonographically guided fine-needle aspiration biopsy of superior mediastinal lesions by the suprasternal route. AJR Am J Roentgenol 1998;171(5):1303–6.
11. Rubens DJ, Strang JG, Fultz PJ, et al. Sonographic guidance of mediastinal biopsy: an effective alternative to CT guidance. AJR Am J Roentgenol 1997; 169(6):1605–10.
12. Petkov R, Minchev T, Yamakova Y, et al. Diagnostic value and complication rate of ultrasound-guided transthoracic core needle biopsy in mediastinal lesions. PloS one 2020;15(4):e0231523.
13. Yang PC, Chang DB, Lee YC, et al. Mediastinal malignancy: ultrasound guided biopsy through the supraclavicular approach. Thorax 1992;47(5): 377–80.
14. Han J, Feng XL, Xu TY, et al. Clinical value of contrast-enhanced ultrasound in transthoracic biopsy of malignant anterior mediastinal masses. J Thorac Dis 2019;11(12):5290–9.
15. Yi D, Feng M, Wen PW, et al. Contrast-enhanced US-guided percutaneous biopsy of anterior mediastinal lesions. Diagn Interv Radiol 2017;23(1):43–8.
16. de Farias AP, Deheinzelin D, Younes RN, et al. Computed tomography-guided biopsy of mediastinal lesions: fine versus cutting needles. Rev Hosp Clin Fac Med Sao Paulo 2003;58(2):69–74.
17. Neema Jamshidi DH, Abtin FG, Loh CT, et al. Genomic adequacy from solid tumor core needle biopsies of ex vivo tissue and in vivo lung masses: prospective study. Radiology 2017; 282(3):903–12.
18. Langen HJ, Klose KC, Keulers P, et al. Artificial widening of the mediastinum to gain access for extrapleural biopsy: clinical results. Radiology 1995; 196(3):703–6.
19. Glassberg RM, Sussman SK, Glickstein MF. CT anatomy of the internal mammary vessels: importance in planning percutaneous transthoracic procedures. AJR Am J Roentgenol 1990;155(2):397–400.
20. Gupta S, Wallace MJ, Morello FA Jr, et al. CT-guided percutaneous needle biopsy of intrathoracic lesions by using the transsternal approach: experience in 37 patients. Radiology 2002;222(1):57–62.
21. Hagberg H, Ahlstrom HK, Magnusson A, et al. Value of transsternal core biopsy in patients with a newly

diagnosed mediastinal mass. Acta Oncol 2000; 39(2):195–8.

22. Astrom KG, Ahlstrom KH, Magnusson A. CT-guided transsternal core biopsy of anterior mediastinal masses. Radiology 1996;199(2):564–7.

23. Belfiore G, Camera L, Moggio G, et al. Middle mediastinum lesions: preliminary experience with CT-guided fine-needle aspiration biopsy with a suprasternal approach. Radiology 1997;202(3):870–3.

24. Gupta S, Seaberg K, Wallace MJ, et al. Imaging-guided percutaneous biopsy of mediastinal lesions: different approaches and anatomic considerations. Radiographics 2005;25(3):763–86 [discussion 786–68].

25. Lal H, Neyaz Z, Nath A, et al. CT-guided percutaneous biopsy of intrathoracic lesions. Korean J Radiol 2012;13(2):210–26.

26. Tantawy WH, El-Gemeie EH, Ibrahim AS, et al. Extrapleural paravertebral CT guided fine needle biopsy of subcarinal lymph nodes. Eur J Radiol 2012;81(10):2907–12.

27. Mills SA, Julian S, Holliday RH, et al. Subxiphoid pericardial window for pericardial effusive disease. J Cardiovasc Surg 1989;30(5):768–73.

28. Yin Z, Liang Z, Li P, et al. CT-guided core needle biopsy of mediastinal nodes through a transpulmonary approach: retrospective analysis of the procedures conducted over six years. Eur Radiol 2017;27(8):3401–7.

29. Bressler EL, Kirkham JA. Mediastinal masses: alternative approaches to CT-guided needle biopsy. Radiology 1994;191(2):391–6.

30. Hiraki T, Kotaro Y, Mimura H, et al. Radiofrequency ablation of metastatic mediastinal lymph nodes during cooling and temperature monitoring of the tracheal mucosa to prevent thermal tracheal damage: initial experience. Radiology 2005;237(3):1068–74.

31. Abtin F, Matthew TQ, Suh R, et al. Percutaneous cryoablation for the treatment of recurrent malignant pleural mesothelioma: safety, early-term efficacy, and predictors of local recurrence. J Vasc Interv Radiol 2017;28(2):213–21.

32. Abtin F, Robert DS, Nasehi L, et al. Percutaneous cryoablation for the treatment of recurrent thymoma:

preliminary safety and efficacy. J Vasc Interv Radiol 2015;26(5):709–14.

33. Arellano RS, Gervais DA, Mueller PR. Computed tomography-guided drainage of mediastinal abscesses: clinical experience with 23 patients. J Vasc Interv Radiol 2011;22(5):673–7.

34. McDermott S, Levis DA, Arellano RS. Chest drainage. Semin Intervent Radiol 2012;29(4):247–55.

35. Maher MM, Lucey BC, Boland G, et al. The role of interventional radiology in the treatment of mediastinal collections caused by esophageal anastomotic leaks. AJR Am J Roentgenol 2002;178(3):649–53.

36. Li L, Zeng XQ, Li YH. CT-guided percutaneous large-needle aspiration and bleomycin sclerotherapy for bronchogenic cyst: report of four cases. J Vasc Interv Radiol 2010;21(7):1045–9.

37. Lakadamyali H, Ergun T, Lakadamyali H, et al. Alcohol ablation therapy of an atypically located symptomatic bronchogenic cyst: a case report. Cardiovasc Intervent Radiol 2007;30(6):1274–6.

38. Heerink WJ, de Bock GH, de Jonge GJ, et al. Complication rates of CT-guided transthoracic lung biopsy: meta-analysis. Eur Radiol 2017;27(1):138–48.

39. Dvorak P, Hoffmann P, Kocova E, et al. CT-guided biopsy of the mediastinal masses. Can anatomical relationships predict complications? Biomed Pap Med Fac Univ Palacky Olomouc Czech Repub 2019;163(3):220–6.

40. Goodacre BW, Savage C, Zwischenberger JB, et al. Salinoma window technique for mediastinal lymph node biopsy. Ann Thorac Surg 2002;74(1):276–7.

41. Lin ZY, Li YG. Artificial pneumothorax with position adjustment for computed tomography-guided percutaneous core biopsy of mediastinum lesions. Ann Thorac Surg 2009;87(3):920–4.

42. Yamagami T, Kato T, Hirota T, et al. Usefulness and limitation of manual aspiration immediately after pneumothorax complicating interventional radiological procedures with the transthoracic approach. Cardiovasc Intervent Radiol 2006;29(6):1027–33.

43. Aquino SDG, Hayman LA. Nerves of the thorax: atlas of normal and pathologic findings. Radiographics 2001;21(5):1275–81.

# Moving?

## Make sure your subscription moves with you!

To notify us of your new address, find your **Clinics Account Number** (located on your mailing label above your name), and contact customer service at:

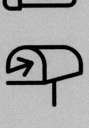

Email: **journalscustomerservice-usa@elsevier.com**

**800-654-2452** (subscribers in the U.S. & Canada)
**314-447-8871** (subscribers outside of the U.S. & Canada)

Fax number: **314-447-8029**

**Elsevier Health Sciences Division**
**Subscription Customer Service**
**3251 Riverport Lane**
**Maryland Heights, MO 63043**

*To ensure uninterrupted delivery of your subscription, please notify us at least 4 weeks in advance of move.

Printed and bound by CPI Group (UK) Ltd, Croydon, CR0 4YY

08/05/2025

01864694-0015